PATIENT SENSE

NEW DIRECTIONS IN RHETORIC AND MATERIALITY
Allison L. Rowland, Christa Teston, and Shui-yin Sharon Yam, Series Editors

PATIENT SENSE

RHETORICAL BODY WORK IN
THE AGE OF TECHNOLOGY

Lillian Campbell

THE OHIO STATE UNIVERSITY PRESS
COLUMBUS

Copyright © 2025 by The Ohio State University.
All rights reserved.

Library of Congress Cataloging-in-Publication Data
Names: Campbell, Lillian (Associate professor of English), author.
Title: Patient sense : rhetorical body work in the age of technology / Lillian Campbell.
Other titles: New directions in rhetoric and materiality.
Description: Columbus : The Ohio State University Press, [2025] | Series: New directions in rhetoric and materiality | Includes bibliographical references and index. | Summary: "Introduces a theory of rhetorical body work and applies it to three sites where care is mediated by new health technologies—a nursing simulation lab, physical therapy lab, and virtual intensive care unit (VICU)—to show how providers' patient sense is maintained and transformed"—Provided by publisher.
Identifiers: LCCN 2025011033 | ISBN 9780814215913 (hardback) | ISBN 0814215912 (hardback) | ISBN 9780814284209 (ebook) | ISBN 0814284205 (ebook)
Subjects: LCSH: Human body—Social aspects. | Medical care—Technological innovations. | Simulated patients. | Virtual reality in medicine.
Classification: LCC HM636 .C36 2025 | DDC 306.4/61—dc23/eng/20250429
LC record available at https://lccn.loc.gov/2025011033

Other identifiers: ISBN 9780814259504 (paperback) | ISBN 0814259502 (paperback)

Cover design by Ashley Muehlbauer
Text design by Juliet Williams
Type set in Adobe Minion Pro

CONTENTS

List of Illustrations		*vii*
INTRODUCTION	The New Healthcare Landscape	1
CHAPTER 1	Rhetorical Body Work	17
CHAPTER 2	A Feeling for the Robot: Embodying Empathy in Nursing Simulations	48
CHAPTER 3	More Than a Massage: Body Work as Boundary-Work in a Physical Therapy Lab	86
CHAPTER 4	Reaching through the Screen: Mediated Body Work in a Virtual Intensive Care Unit	124
CONCLUSION	Body Matters for the Future of Healthcare and Technology	161
Acknowledgments		*171*
Appendix 1	*Nursing Simulation Interview Questions*	*175*
Appendix 2	*Physical Therapy Interview Questions*	*179*
Appendix 3	*Tele-Observation Interview Questions*	*182*
Works Cited		*185*
Index		*195*

ILLUSTRATIONS

FIGURE 1	Several nursing students provide care for a male robotic patient	58
FIGURE 2	Interpersonal patient information charted by students	80
TABLE 1	Overview of tele-observer study participants	134

INTRODUCTION

The New Healthcare Landscape

Technological innovations are rapidly changing the landscape of healthcare. As a patient, you might see this when you visit the doctor and try to hold their attention while they click through pages upon pages of electronic charting (Gawande). You might be adjusting to virtual appointments with some of your providers or navigating the dynamics of a therapy appointment over video call (Bedor Hiland). You might even be noticing that supervisors at work are making new kinds of arguments about your health, ones that rely on algorithmic predictions based on biometric data points (Graham; Stambler). As patients, we can account for the ways these technological changes influence our interactions with providers—toward fewer physical interactions of body on body, fewer moments of connection, maybe even less conversation altogether. But what do these shifts mean for the training of new healthcare practitioners and the future of their professional roles?

Indeed, new technologies are transforming the embodied work of future healthcare providers, necessitating new kinds of patient interaction and at times calling into question a profession's role in patient care. When nurses can complete portions of their clinical hours with robotic patients, and medical assistants might spend their entire careers providing patient care mediated by a screen, their understanding and embodiment of their roles must change. Rhetoric is at the heart of this education as future providers learn how to communicate with their patients and reframe their understanding of expertise in collaboration with a range of new technologies.

This book takes up these transformations in embodied professional practice in three allied health professions—nursing, physical therapy, and tele-observation. I introduce a theory of rhetorical body work to frame the embodied shifts that are occurring in response to technological mediation of patient care. In addition, I foreground the concept of patient sense to account for the intuitive patient knowledge that providers leverage in their care and advocacy for patients.

Drawing on sociological frameworks (Gimlin), I define rhetorical body work as paid physical, emotional, and/or discursive labor performed at the material or technological interface of worker–client bodies. Sociological theories of body work emphasize how it is devalued within social and institutional systems and often gendered and racialized (Wolkowitz, *Bodies*). Fields with professional prestige, like medicine, maintain that prestige through limiting bodily contact and cordoning off bodily parts (Wolkowitz, "Social Relations" 501). Meanwhile, patient sense, a corollary to Beverly Sauer's "pit sense" in her research on risk communication in mining, captures the complex embodied knowledge that informs health practitioners' care. Patient sense is acquired through extended encounters with bodies as providers build their expertise over time and in a range of contexts. Rhetorical scholars will recognize patient sense as a type of embodied *phronesis,* or practical wisdom, that is specific to clinical contexts and healthcare.

To truly study the embodied practices of providers, those practices must be observed in situ through sustained fieldwork in professional settings. Thus, this book draws on ethnographic fieldwork and interviews with focal participants at three sites—a nursing simulation lab, a physical therapy lab, and a virtual intensive care unit (VICU). I leverage a multimodal methodology that included video recordings alongside participant accounts to capture and analyze embodied learning and practices. Drawing on these rich data sets, this book uncovers the complex embodied, emotional, and discursive work that providers offer across contexts, even as they interface with and mediate care through new technologies.

These technologies transform the rhetorical body work that healthcare providers must learn, and yet the technologies do not replace the empathetic knowledge that undergirds their interactions, the professional knowledge and embodied expertise that shapes their practice, or the intuitive cues that inform their interventions. As much as this book acknowledges and accounts for the important role of technology in transforming our healthcare landscape, it also centers human bodies in interaction with one another. Ultimately, I argue that we will always need responsive expert healthcare providers whose rhetorical body work cannot be replaced by technicians or algorithms.

Technological Transformations in Healthcare

Before delving into the specifics of my framework, I contextualize this project within three national trends: (1) the ubiquity of simulations in the education of healthcare providers, (2) the rise in virtual patient care and remote patient monitoring during COVID-19, and (3) the spread of AI technology in patient diagnosis and care. These three transitions mark an important moment for considering the precarity of health professionals in the future, as workers that center body-on-body action transition to technology-mediated contexts.

Simulation Education

Did you know that your healthcare provider probably first practiced palpating a patient's abdomen on a life-sized robotic manikin?[1] Are you aware that the first baby your obstetric nurse helped deliver might very well have been Baby Hal, a robot? Clinical simulations are ubiquitous in the health professions, and most community colleges and universities that train health professionals have some version of a simulation lab. However, after conducting my research on clinical nursing simulations, I discovered that for those outside of healthcare education, clinical simulation remains largely unknown. This is an important oversight because patient simulations have a prominent role in shaping the way that medical professionals come to interpret and articulate the body. In other words, they have become part of the landscape of "technocorporality": "the ways in which technologies are becoming (or perhaps, were always) entwined with our bodies, experiences, and existences" (Sundén 97).

While early prototyping of simulation manikins began as early as 1963 at the University of Southern California, it was not until 2000, when Laerdal introduced the first "SimMan"—their brand name for their robotic manikin—that simulation technology became financially viable for most medical training programs. Now, simulated manikins are used extensively in practitioner training programs for nurses, doctors, anesthesiologists, and others (Rosen 162).[2] Simulations in healthcare education today can take many different forms, including the use of plastic model parts that mimic the feel of particular practices as well as the use of patient educators—actors or trained volunteers who can offer feedback to doctors in training.[3] Sara Press's research on the rhetoric of standardized patient programs during the twentieth century demonstrates how programs have grappled with "how to represent a

---

   1. "Manikin" is the preferred terminology to describe full-body patient simulators in healthcare contexts. "Mannequin" is thought to be affiliated with fashion contexts.
   2. The year 2000 also marked the release of the Institute of Medicine's report "To Err Is Human: Building a Safer Health System," which reported that 44,000 to 98,000 Americans were dying each year from preventable medical errors. The report proposed extending simulation training as one direction for improvement.
   3. Nonfiction writer Leslie Jamison has written about her experiences working as a patient actor in the aptly titled essay "Empathy Exams."

biomedical disease *and* a patient group while retaining the individuality of a single patient" (308). Her research points to one of the ongoing challenges in healthcare training more broadly, which is that often to teach cultural sensitivity, programs lean into generalizations or stereotypes about populations. This can ultimately counter their goals by reinforcing problematic assumptions about certain groups.

Despite their ubiquity, simulation experiences are rarely seen as a complete replacement for clinical experience and instead are positioned as a supplement that can provide students with hands-on practice prior to and during their interactions with live patients (Nehring and Lashley). In addition, simulations are valued for providing opportunities for students to act in high-risk situations that they may not encounter during their short time in clinical environments, as well as for the ability to debrief with instructors and peers after interactions.

Still, research in gender studies and science studies has been critical of the SimMan manikins that are a focal feature of many simulation labs. Johnson has argued that robotic manikins perpetuate one-sex body models "in which female is a subset of male" (155). Meanwhile, Sundén describes the gendered and racialized limitations of "blonde birth machines" that because they are "routinely portrayed and sold as white" enable students and instructors to efface race in their care (110). She argues that adding details like hair and breasts to birthing simulators but not the fluids, odors, or sounds that accompany birthing represents a "selective bodily awareness" that supports problematic gender conceptions in the medical imagination (107). However, both authors are also aware of the limitations of studying patient simulators as static objects outside of their context of use. Similarly, the rhetorical body work approach that frames this project calls for attention to how simulation manikins and environments shape student interactions, informing their understanding and performance of embodied and empathetic patient care.

Telehealth

Definitions of telehealth vary, but most focus on the presence of mediating technologies to support communication either between providers (like the electronic health record) or between provider and patient (like a video call). A subset of telehealth, telemedicine describes the delivery of medical care through communication technologies like laptops, smartphones, tablets, and so forth (Bedor Hiland 112). In my first two case studies, providers are still delivering care face-to-face with patients, while using technologies to mediate that care and their communication with other providers—telehealth. My final site features telemedicine, the delivery of healthcare via video cameras and microphones.

While telehealth's widespread use in hospitals and clinical contexts is relatively new, most historians identify 1959 as its beginning in the United States, when the Nebraska Psychiatric Institute and Norfolk State Hospital in Nebraska used microwave television to communicate and conduct research (Breen and Matusitz). Meanwhile, one of the National Aeronautics and Space Administration's first areas of research and development was designing astronaut suits that would constantly measure physiological data and share it using communication satellites, an early telehealth technology. In the late 1960s and early 1970s, the federal government invested in applying these monitoring technologies to rural areas, such as a program developed for the Papago people in southern Arizona (Breen and Matusitz). The 1970s also saw the use of telehealth technologies in the Navy to monitor and support crew members' weight loss from afar (Florea et al. 319). Overall, as telecommunication technology has evolved, telehealth's possibilities have expanded, but it was still often "categorized, niche-oriented, and narrowed down to provide specific services for particular sectors, contexts and applications" (Breen and Matusitz 62).

However, the COVID-19 pandemic created an impetus for widespread integration and adoption of telemedicine on a very condensed timeline, engaging skeptics from both the professional and patient spheres. Telemedicine made up a very small part of healthcare operations until 2020, when its reimbursement and licensure rules were temporarily changed due to the pandemic. A March 2023 report from the Office of the National Coordinator for Health Information Technology tracked a rapid shift from 15 percent of office-based physicians using any form of telemedicine in 2018–19 to an increase to 87 percent in 2021.

In her book on tele-mental healthcare, Bedor Hiland describes her experiences with teletherapy shortly after the start of the pandemic. While both she and her provider had previously disparaged virtual services, several weeks into the pandemic Bedor Hiland discovered that her provider had started using an online platform, prioritizing continuance of care over discomfort with virtual sessions. While Bedor Hiland found the virtual experience "diluted, depersonalized, and even surreal" (139), it also offered an outlet for therapy at a time of high stress and need. Thus, COVID-19 created an exigency for many providers and patients, sometimes begrudgingly, to integrate telemedicine into their practice.

Despite its relatively rapid adoption, telehealth still receives frequent critiques, especially when telehealth professionals are integrated alongside practitioners on the hospital floor. For example, studies of staff acceptance of telehealth show that workers tend to be resistant to the experience of being monitored by tele-ICU staff (Stafford et al.; Moeckli et al.). In addition, communication breakdowns often occur because practitioners continue to rely on prior chains of command even when tele-experts are present (Moeckli et al.). Sand-Jecklin et al. similarly found disconnects between nurses and virtual monitoring technicians (VMTs) in their interviews. Nurses were more likely to blame VMT distraction as central to errors, while VMTs blamed slow nurse response and problems with the technology and complained about nurses not always participating in patient hand-offs (147–48). In addition, because hospitals often use algorithms to decide which patients should receive virtual monitoring, telehealth is vulnerable to algorithmic bias and design flaws that I discuss in the next section as well (Noble; Benjamin).

Algorithms and Patient Care

Together with the transition toward telehealth is the integration of algorithms into patient monitoring and care. As Graham explains in his book *The Doctor and the Algorithm,* the early 2020s represented a moment of Artificial Intelligence "summer" during which there was great enthusiasm and optimism about the potential for AI integration to transform the landscape of healthcare. This was accompanied by a "proliferation of health AI focused on diagnosis, prognosis, healthcare systems management, drug discovery, disease modeling, and so on" (4). In *Deep Medicine,* Topol argues that the integration of AI into burdensome tasks like charting in electronic medical records or analyzing lab results might increase opportunities for patient interaction and emotional connection. Indeed, medical providers have critiqued the increased burdens of charting with the advent of electronic health records and offered up integration of AI-based documenting as one possible solution (Gawande).

Of course, given widespread research that demonstrates the shortcomings of AI and its propensity to reproduce social inequities (Noble; Benjamin), many are skeptical of its positive impact. Prior research in fields like law has provided a glimpse into the disastrous effects of inaccurate and bias-laden AI recommendations in critical applications, with impacts including exacerbated poverty (Macaulay), wrongful arrest (George et al.), and unjust criminal sentencing (Holzinger et al.).

It is undeniable, however, that AI is demonstrating it can outperform human practitioners in certain types of medical tasks, especially diagnosis. In 2020 an AI system exceeded the performance of human cardiologists in

ECG-based diagnosis (Siontis et al.). Meanwhile, in 2023 a study reported that AI-supported mammogram screening increased breast cancer detection by 20 percent (Lång et al.). As a result, some hospital systems are buying big into AI in the hopes that it will have widespread impacts, reducing medical error and mortality rates. For example, in 2019 a large academic medical system in southeastern Wisconsin implemented the Rothman Index, a patient-deterioration algorithm designed by Perahealth that uses nurses' documentation in patient charts to calculate the likelihood of patient decline and alert practitioners. The implementation of the Rothman was, in fact, the impetus for my research team to begin studying the virtual intensive care unit that I describe in chapter 4, though by the time we began our research the contract with Perahealth had already ended.

Our retrospective interviews with doctors and administrators at the hospital identified several conflicts with and critiques of the Rothman system, including its reliance on nurses' documentation, which was frequently delayed, and its overly sensitive alert system, which meant that doctors quickly learned to ignore alarms. On a more fundamental level, many of our interviewees were unwilling to accept the assumption that an algorithm could exceed a trained professional with years of experience at predicting patient decline; they resented the hospital's large financial commitment to this assumption (Campbell et al.). Similar research on perceptions of early warning algorithms has found nearly identical challenges to our study, including limitations related to provider buy-in (Foley and Dowling), delays in documentation (Watson et al.), and warning fatigue, which is often coupled with decreased compliance (Cooper et al.; Bailey et al.).

On the other hand, attitudes toward the Rothman differed when we spoke to nurses in the VICU. From their perspective, the Rothman offered the advantage of regular opportunities for communication with nurses on the hospital floor. As the director of the VICU explained, without the Rothman alerts, VICU staff did not always have reasons for outreach to floor personnel, which limited their ability to hold practitioners accountable and advocate for patients. The director also noted that relationships with practitioners on the floor are "always a little dicey." The team had been working to develop a consultative and mentoring relationship with floor nurses, especially new hires, and in that way the Rothman aligned with their goals. Positioning themselves as a resource for new nurses helped the VICU nurses to develop a more collaborative relationship, while also enabling them to provide support and accountability for those who are most in need (Campbell et al.). This aligns with findings that healthcare workers are more willing to accept the use of technology in their workplace when they see benefits for themselves (e.g., time reduction, improvement of relations), or what are sometimes called complementarity effects (Wang et al.).

Throughout the duration of our research in the VICU, my research team and I also noted a transition away from deterioration indexes like Rothman and toward algorithm-enabled wellness technologies. As it ended its contract with Perahealth, the hospital network in our study also implemented several remote patient monitoring and patient telehealth programs using AI-enabled wellness technologies for COVID-19 recovery, prenatal health, and mental health. These tools relied on data provided by patients either through direct input or home monitoring technologies, thereby overcoming some of the limitations of algorithmic systems that primarily use nurses' documentation. Of course, this introduces new limitations as well, such as the racial biases of oximeter technology, which featured centrally in COVID-19 monitoring (Graham 13).

Rhetorical Body Work: Learning, Communicating, and Valuing Patient Sense

Having established three key elements in the current technological healthcare landscape, I move now into introducing my theoretical framework for this project—rhetorical body work—and the related concept of patient sense. I first encountered the sociological concept of body work when I was writing about gendered learning in nursing simulations (Campbell, "Simulating Gender") and read Fisher's study of body-work strategies among male nurses in Australia. Drawing on interviews with twenty-one Australian male nurses, Fisher describes the various physical and emotional strategies they use to navigate their gendered positioning during care in a field that is frequently feminized. These include reading patient body language and tone; modifying their physical interactions, especially touch; and bringing in witnesses to the scene. Fisher's study captured exactly the kind of embodied and emotional disciplinary practices that I was so interested in studying in my own research. By extension, I turned to this sociological framework and found it rich, especially for how it articulates an intersection between workplace practices and physiological experiences of the body including touch, smell, sight, and even taste.

Body work offers a unique approach for considering embodied training in professional disciplines because it situates specific embodied learning and practices within economic networks of exchange. Theories of body work link the smile that a nurse teaches herself to provide while experiencing disgust to a labor market that puts a price on her emotional performances (Wolkowitz,

"Social Relations"). Body work simultaneously calls attention to how power is distributed by distancing oneself from embodied interactions and how the most bodily labor is often reserved for the most vulnerable populations, especially women of color. It forces us not to ignore the racial hierarchies that separate so many of us from the products of our bodies and that relegate bodily work to individuals who often remain invisible. Overall, to talk about embodied rhetorics in workplace contexts without a view of their economic valuing and relationship to stratified hierarchies is to overlook a key aspect of professionals' rhetorical work.

Meanwhile, I initially introduced the concept of patient sense while analyzing my fieldwork in clinical nursing simulations and engaging with Sauer's ("Embodied Knowledge") ethnographic research on embodied communication in the mining industry (Campbell, *Simulating Nursing* 187). Sauer's study demonstrates how communicative impasses emerge between miners who rely on physical, intuitive knowledge about the mines and scientists and engineers who use professional tools and technical documentation to ensure miners' safety. Based on these distinctions, Sauer established three categories of expertise—pit sense, engineering experience, and scientific knowledge. These categories describe a spectrum of expertise that begins with direct physical interaction with the environment and extends to the advanced interpretation of mediated data drawing on professional scientific knowledge.

When my colleague Elizabeth Angeli and I began coding data from emergency medical service providers and nursing students to account for the role of intuition in patient care, we again turned to the concept of patient sense to describe the embodied sensory knowledge that health providers gain from physical presence alongside and in contact with the patient (Angeli and Campbell, "Intuition"). However, as our research developed, our focus shifted, and we ultimately introduced a taxonomy of sensory cues that prompt embodied intuition and did not include patient sense (Campbell and Angeli). As I brought together the case studies in this project, I realized I needed a concept to capture the intuitive, embodied knowledge that was so central to the learning and practice of my providers. Thus, I returned to patient sense and unpacked its relationship to rhetorical body work.

Rhetorical scholars will likely recognize connections between patient sense and the ancient Greek concept of phronesis, or practical wisdom. Scholars describe phronesis as a praxis that bridges everyday skills and techniques (techne) and theory (theoria), contextualizing our moment-by-moment actions within larger ethical aims (Smith 88). Previous scholars have connected phronesis to healthcare contexts, defining it as clinical judgment and arguing that practitioners use phronesis to "combine scientific information, clinical skill, and collective experience" to develop a plan for patient care (Montgomery 5). Relevant to my contexts, Rentmeester et al. argue for the importance of phronesis to physical therapists' negotiation of patient care ("Hermeneutical Healing") and to nurses' transitions from novice to expert provider ("Gadamerian Approach").

While phronesis has at times been described as the more disembodied and socially acceptable corollary to the concept of *métis* (Dolmage 11), rhetoricians of health and medicine have also reclaimed its embodied qualities, especially for healthcare practitioners (Teston 178; Campbell and Angeli 374). In chapter 1, I delve more deeply into these conversations to consider both phronesis and métis in relationship to embodied rhetoric, ethics, and education. For now, I position patient sense under the larger umbrella of phronesis, as a type of contextualized and embodied patient knowledge that enables providers to navigate between their abstract understanding of medicine and their response to individual patients with unique experiences.

Patient sense is a specific type of phronesis that plays a unique role in learning, engaging, and communicating body work. First, since all three of my chapters are invested in understanding how newcomers learn the embodied, emotional, and discursive strategies of their future fields, I recognize patient sense as a key component of the professional body work that students are acquiring. For example, in nursing simulations, instructors manipulate the simulation environment and the manikin patient to replicate clinical environments and cue students' intuitive patient knowledge. Whether they are using a warm rice pack to mimic a blood clot or green Vaseline to look like an infected wound, simulations are designed to help students acquire patient sense to both practice relevant body work and prepare for future care. While the patient bodies look different, the attention to acquisition of embodied, intuitive patient knowledge is similar in physical therapy labs as well, while the tele-observers' patient sense drew on a wide range of professional and educational experiences.

In addition, professionals in these three fields necessarily must find ways to communicate their patient sense to others both within and across disciplines. Sauer's research argues that translating pit sense poses a unique challenge given that this knowledge is experienced "as physical signs or sensations in [miners'] bodies" and is rarely discursive ("Embodied Knowledge" 134). She demonstrates how embodied knowledge often shows up as gestures rather than language in retrospective interviews ("Embodied Experience"). Similarly, health providers use rhetorical body work, including a range of emotional, physical, and discursive strategies, to translate their patient sense to others. These strategies range from nursing students adding a note section to their chart about a patient's emotional state to tele-observers' leveraging interpersonal alliances to elevate their patient sense in conversations and ensure their perspectives are valued.

Finally, as members of allied health professions, nursing, physical therapy, and tele-observation professionals all struggle to maintain legitimacy and to argue for their unique expertise specifically because they are fields that center the body and patient sense. Rhetorical body work plays a key role in framing their work and creating a hierarchy of desirability for bodily jobs (i.e., massage therapist vs. sex worker; certified nursing assistant vs. nurse). Patient sense is critical to this negotiation. First, because it runs counter to biomedical perspectives of health that foreground quantifiable metrics and data. And second, because for all three professions, their holistic approach to patient care that foregrounds understanding unique patient experiences is part of what distinguishes them from others. Thus, rhetorical body work is used to establish professional expertise and argue for the legitimacy of patient sense as a complement to biomedical understanding. For example, physical therapists learn to use embodied and emotional moves in their patient care that act as boundary-work, both by masculinizing their profession and by highlighting their scientific expertise.

Researching Bodies at Work

With these intersections between rhetorical body work and patient sense in mind, my analysis is guided by a focus on professional practices, technological mediation, and distribution of power. Across my varied research contexts, I ask:

- What embodied, emotional, and discursive practices are prioritized and taught in each allied health profession, and how is that body work tied to their professional histories and identities?
- How does technological mediation of patient sense and embodied cues transform the work of patient care?
- In what ways do the gendered and racialized biases associated with rhetorical body work and patient sense change in new professional and technological contexts?

To answer those questions, this book's argument is built on three richly developed ethnographic data sets in three different allied health professional contexts, drawing on fieldwork that has been conducted over the past decade.

Data includes over one hundred hours of observation on-site and over seventy-five interviews, in addition to dozens of documents. While research on embodied rhetoric is prevalent, this expansive multimodal data set is both unique and necessary given the goals of the project. And as I will demonstrate, all three sites speak to a number of the changes described above through their involvement in training healthcare students to work with future health technologies.

Another unique contribution of this book is my focus on educational sites, where students are learning professional practices and embodiment for the first time. Educational contexts are an ideal site for research on body work because disciplinary practices that will later become tacit and entrenched are openly identified and discussed with newcomers. For example, nursing simulations featured debriefs during which instructors and students would reflect together on strengths and limitations of the group's interactions with a robotic patient. In workplace contexts, this explicit reflection on communication is unlikely due to time constraints. In addition, educational contexts are particularly valuable for studying the intersections between gender, race, bodies, and work. As Hallenbeck and Smith argue, "Sites of education are powerful loci within which students develop an intellectual and physical habitus, and thus often serve to naturalize gendered, classed, and raced relations" (214). All my contexts featured moments where power relations were made explicit for learners who have yet to fully accept and embody them.

While the contexts for my research had significant differences and my methods varied in response, my research designs shared several features. First, all three projects were approved by the human subject board at my institution and the institution where they took place. In line with this human subjects approval, I use pseudonyms throughout to refer to students, instructors, workers, and research sites. All the projects included observations of a full cohort of students or workers. To conduct those observations, I distributed consent forms to all students or workers; anyone who opted out was not included in my field notes or analysis, though they may have inadvertently been captured in video recordings. All three projects also included interviews with a smaller group of students or workers who opted into participating in the study further during the initial consent phase for a small stipend. I refer to this group as focal participants or focal students.

I did have significant variations in the number of focal students and interviews conducted at each site. The nursing simulation study included five focal students and four interviews each, an introductory interview and one after each of three simulations during their sophomore year (see appendix 1). The physical therapy study included twenty-nine focal students and two interviews each, an introductory interview and a reflective interview after my classroom recording of their care (see appendix 2). The VICU study included seven focal participants and one interview each, following my on-site observations (see appendix 3). At all three sites, I also collected relevant documents including student writing and various forms of documentation.

A key difference between my sites was the degree to which I was able to video record participants. The clinical nursing simulations already included a video recording system so that students who were not participating in a simulation could watch it from another room. Instructors kept copies of all the simulation recordings on file in their main office. With student consent, I copied the recordings of the simulations and then had easy access to high-quality color footage. Student debriefs with their instructors after the simulations were not recorded, however, so I attended these and took field notes on the conversations. By contrast, there was no existing recording system in the physical technologies lab where I observed physical therapy students. Therefore, I brought my own tripod and video camera and could only record one small group of two to three students interacting at a time. In chapter 3, I elaborate on how I made decisions about who to record. In both cases, I ended with approximately thirty hours of video data. Meanwhile, due to patient privacy restrictions in the virtual intensive care unit, I was not able to record interactions in that space but did conduct twenty hours of field observations.

In chapter 1, I elaborate on what I call the "ethnographic perspective" of this research drawing on current research on rhetorical field methods. Broadly, my presence on-site supported my inquiry into the material experiences of both the researcher and research subjects and provided me a more comprehensive understanding of my sites as unique and vibrant rhetorical contexts. To make this visible in my analysis, each body chapter features a "My Body on the Scene" section where I describe a brief period during field observations where my own embodiment and experience of the research site was foregrounded.[4] While I realize that these excerpts cannot fully account for the impact of my body and positionality on the analysis presented, I hope that by including them early in each chapter I can acknowledge my embodied influence on this research without detracting from the perspectives of my participants, whose voices I work to center.

Since questions about access and interdisciplinary collaboration are often raised in rhetoric of health and medicine scholarship, I also include some details about how I gained access to my research sites in each of my body

---

4. Elizabeth Angeli's "Scene Size-Ups" in her book on rhetoric in emergency medical services offered me a model for these sections.

chapters. Here I will simply mention that it is no mistake that conducting fieldwork at three separate healthcare sites took over a decade. Each site required years of investment and relationship-building, and for every successful collaboration, I had dozens of conversations with potential collaborators that did not become projects. This investment of time and energy is tied to my firm belief in the value of richly contextualized qualitative research in rhetoric of health and medicine. I think we can learn things from studying communication in situ that we cannot possibly learn just from looking at texts or conducting retrospective interviews. And while I recognize the time commitment and challenges that accompany such fieldwork, I also hope to encourage those who may be in the process to keep initiating conversations and pursuing avenues for access.

Overview of the Book

The book proceeds first by setting a theoretical groundwork—introducing the concepts of rhetorical body work and patient sense—and then examining each of my research sites through that framework. Chapter 1, "Rhetorical Body Work," overviews rhetorical body-work research from both sociology and rhetoric of health and medicine and connects it to the concept of patient sense. I argue that sociological perspectives offer material rhetoricians a framework for better attending to the body/work nexus in ways that emphasize power relationships between individuals and connect workplace hierarchies to larger systems of racialized and gendered oppression. Meanwhile, rhetoricians taking up the rhetorical body can be particularly attuned to the role that language plays in the teaching and performance of body work. I conclude this chapter with methodological reflections on studying rhetorical body work in situ, expanding on the brief methodological discussions provided above.

Chapter 2, "A Feeling for the Robot," draws on my fieldwork in clinical nursing simulations to consider whether robots can teach patient-centered care. I begin by outlining intersections between research on simulation and empathy, considering how the theoretical framework of body work enriches both conversations. Then, I analyze embodied, emotional, and discursive learning in my observations and recordings of clinical nursing simulations, working through several saliant examples to demonstrate the extent to which patient sense and rhetorical body work are taught and reinforced through human–machine interaction. Central to my argument is the importance of disruption in simulations. Simulations are disruptive because they cannot perfectly replicate patient sense in clinical contexts, but that disruption serves a critical role by supporting student responsiveness and reflection. I conclude with a rare but troublesome scene from one of the simulations that points to the risks of empathetic learning, especially in instances where cultural differences between the patient and student are foregrounded. This raises questions about the limitations of pedagogies of empathy and points to the need for strategies that can help students grapple with difference without devolving into disengagement.

Chapter 3, "More Than a Massage," draws on my fieldwork in the physical therapy lab to better understand how pedagogies of body work are tied to professional identity and ethos. I describe the precarious disciplinary positioning of "touch professions," caused in part by their proximity to the body and reliance on patient sense. Then, I show how instructors in physical therapy counter gendered associations with body work as feminine, sexualized, and nonexpert. First, I consider the stories that circulate in the lab, which simultaneously work to highlight the scientific expertise of physical therapy professionals and to demonstrate strategies for creating physical boundaries to desexualize the patient encounter. Next, I describe physical learning in the lab—both body-on-body contact and technology-mediated care—to describe how students acquire patient sense alongside embodied practices that emphasize their expertise and unique knowledge base. I demonstrate how both the stories that circulate and the embodied lessons in the lab run the risk of reinforcing patient stereotypes and gendered assumptions about professionalism. Thus, this chapter also attends to the hidden curriculum of these embodied lessons and consequences for patient care.

Finally, chapter 4, "Reaching through the Screen," unpacks the patient sense and communication practices that workers from a wide range of professional backgrounds bring to tele-observation and questions how technological mediation changes the nature of their body work. Tele-observers' primary job is virtual patient monitoring. From a remote location, they are responsible for watching and listening to six to eight high-risk patients on a large double screen and alerting hospital staff if the patients break protocol. Undoubtedly, body work in tele-observation is still racialized and gendered—most of my interview participants were Black women. It is still clearly marginalized— low-paid, with little professional training or support. However, the conversations I had with tele-observers demonstrated how they leverage patient sense gained in a range of educational and professional contexts as well as from their knowledge of new technologies. Meanwhile, they rely on complex emotional negotiations with other providers to ensure that their patient sense is valued and legitimized. This final analysis chapter argues for greater attention to marginalized care workers' professional histories as well as recognition of the important role their bodies play even in mediated patient care.

My conclusion synthesizes findings across research sites to argue for the vital role of healthcare pedagogy in preparing students for the physical, emotional, and discursive work that will accompany their future roles. I attend to the specific disciplinary lessons in body work that are occurring in nursing, physical therapy, and tele-observation and how those lessons are tied to their professional histories and identities. In addition, I consider the impact of technological mediation on patient sense and how gendered and racialized biases associated with rhetorical body work transform in new technological contexts. My discussion points to the potential for professional precarity in these fields as technologies infiltrate everyday practice and patient care.

Overall, by bringing the lens of body work to rhetorical scholarship, this book offers a groundwork for future research that investigates the relationships between individuals' embodied and discursive action and global systems of economic exchange. At the same time, a rhetorical approach to body work emphasizes its interactive and persuasive nature in ways that have been overlooked in sociological scholarship, including how embodied exchanges between practitioner and patient are discursively captured and communicated. By connecting these theoretical interventions to a kairotic moment where technology is shaping all aspects of patient care, this book intervenes into what is guaranteed to be ongoing conversations about the future of healthcare training. My case studies demonstrate the ongoing need for rhetorically responsive providers whose embodied expertise cannot be replaced by technicians or algorithms.

CHAPTER 1

Rhetorical Body Work

Throughout this book, I define rhetorical body work as paid physical, emotional, or discursive labor performed at the material or technological interface of worker–client bodies. In this chapter, I deconstruct different components of that definition to identify their theoretical origins as well as contemporary debates. I also highlight the role that patient sense plays in relation to rhetorical body work, especially during its acquisition, translation, and valuing. My definition draws heavily on research in sociology, where the concept of body work originated. Specifically, my emphasis on paid labor—as opposed to care work or the management of personal relationships—draws on sociological framing. Below, I also integrate scholarship on the relationship between work and labor to contextualize my discussions of work.

Similarly, my attention to the intersection of physical and emotional labor speaks to two of the four sociological approaches to body work that Gimlin describes in her review of research on body work—body work/labor and body/emotional management. Sociologist Carol Wolkowitz's book, *Bodies at Work*, focuses on the first nexus, body work/labor, by considering how the circulation of body work reinforces class stratification along racialized and gendered lines (*Bodies*). For example, female immigrants often take on the most physical tasks as nursing assistants or nail technicians. Meanwhile, Hochschild's research on emotional management considers the second category, body/emotion management, through Hochschild's attention to how employees produce or suppress emotions, like the demand that waitresses always be smiling in front of customers (*Managed Heart*). Overall, I argue that sociological perspectives offer rhetoricians a framework for better attending to the body/work nexus in ways that emphasize power relationships between individuals and connect professional hierarchies to larger systems of racialized and gendered oppression. In my review of scholarship, I integrate feminist and disability studies perspectives as well, to attend to differing definitions of the body.

At the same time, my discussions of discursive labor are unique, integrating a rhetorical framework into prior scholarship on body work. While there is a wide range of research on rhetorics of the body, I home in on a more limited conversation that is focused on embodied communication in professional contexts with particular attention to the teaching of these embodied practices. I also discuss approaches to studying rhetoric in situ, drawing on rhetorical field-methods frameworks and outlining my ethnographic approach to the three case studies in this book. Bringing these perspectives together, I demonstrate how rhetoricians taking up the rhetorical body can be particularly attuned to discourse's role in the teaching and performance of body work and the communication of patient sense. I offer methodological considerations for anyone interested in similar research.

In addition, a major contribution of this book is its consideration of how body work and patient sense both transform and remain consistent when they are mediated through a variety of technologies. To attend to mediated patient sense and body work, I draw on research on material rhetorics and object-oriented theories in this chapter as well. These perspectives provide initial framing for the book's larger argument that technologies transform the rhetorical body work of healthcare providers but do not replace it. New healthcare technologies do not eliminate the need for empathetic patient knowledge that shapes nurses' communication; the professional knowledge and expertise that informs a physical therapist's touch; or the intuitive bodily cues that inform tele-observers' interventions. Thus, just as my definition of rhetorical body work centers worker and patient bodies, this book maintains a focus on human bodies in interaction with one another despite its attention to technological mediation. The sociological origins of body work help to keep that human perspective in focus, even as I bring a wide range of embodied and material frameworks into conversation.

Origins of Body Work

Why does research on the body tend to focus on the home, public spaces, or extracurricular activities? Why do we so rarely consider the body in workplace contexts? In her article "The Social Relations of Body Work," Wolkowitz posed these questions for the field of sociology, setting out the premise for a new framework that avoids relegating the body to extracurricular contexts and instead brings embodiment back into the focus in workplace studies. She explained: "Until fairly recently, sociologists seemed to agree that where the body is, work is not. [. . .] We associate sensuousness with play, desire and spontaneity, rather than with employment's numbing routines" (498). Wolkowitz is often considered one of the founders of body work, along with Gimlin, whose 2002 book *Body Work: Beauty and Self-Image in American Culture* was contemporaneous with Wolkowitz's article. While the two take a shared interest in the overlap between economic systems and bodily labor, Wolkowitz's focus on physical work and emotional labor for employees on the job aligns more closely with my framework, as opposed to Gimlin's focus on the work of maintaining physical appearances.

Both Wolkowitz and Gimlin have argued that the field of sociology tends to overlook the nexus between work and the body. On the one hand, while sociological research on work in the 1920s to the 1930s attended to the embodied and emotional experiences of workers, it also contrasted these with the rational, disembodied approach of managers, already equating body work with working-class labor, a theme I discuss in more detail later in this chapter (Gimlin, "What Is Body Work?" 354). On the other hand, Wolkowitz argues that some feminist sociological research on the body was part of a cultural turn that led to a perspective of the body as shaped by cultural consumption rather than as an active force of its own (*Bodies* 18). Thus, Wolkowitz has called for a shift from social constructionist approaches to the body. She argues instead that we should contextualize the body's formation as part of "routinized workplace encounters, mediated by the cash nexus, and located within wider social inequalities" ("Social Relations" 505). This definition resonates with several perspectives in rhetoric and disability studies as well that have argued that scholars overemphasize signification of the body and body as signifier while undervaluing the body's active role in moment-by-moment rhetorical action (Kerschbaum; Kessler).

Work

Of course, one cannot discount a rich history of philosophers and sociologists engaging with questions of body work. In fact, in her call back to the body for sociologists of work, Wolkowitz notes that the field has been "conveniently forgetting Marx's realization that people can only remake their bodies through labor" ("Social Relations" 498). Indeed, Marxist scholarship elaborates on distinctions between categories like labor, work, and care, importantly setting parameters on how one might define work's relationship to the body. Both

Arendt and Fraser, for example, parse the differences between labor and work, attributing the former to activities that pertain directly to bodily sustenance and existence and the latter to the production of objects that have use-value within a capitalist economy. Arendt argues that labor exists "to produce whatever is necessary to keep the human organism alive" and work "to create whatever is needed to house the human body" (29). She notes that most languages distinguish between labor and work and that "in all these cases, the equivalents for labor have an unequivocal connotation of bodily experiences, of toil, and troubles, and in most cases, they are significantly also used for the pangs of birth" (32).

Concomitant with labor's direct connection to embodied experience is the fact that its timing corresponds with the life cycle, beginning with birth and ending with death, rather than culminating in the production of a specific object for use. Fabrication and usage are also not separately defined occurrences, as they are in the case of work, so the alienation from material production that characterizes Marxist frameworks is less evident in discussions of labor. Or as Arendt explains, "The blessing of labor is that effort and gratification follow each other as closely as producing and consuming, so that happiness is a concomitant of the process itself" (34). This sense of gratification should not be confused, she argues, with the brief happiness of completing an object that occurs during work processes.

Fifty years later, Fraser takes up Marxist frameworks to consider the background conditions of economic systems, especially the labor of care. Much like Arendt's distinctions between work and labor, Fraser highlights the ways that devalued labor is also the most closely tied to embodied experience: "'Care,' 'affective labour' or 'subjectivation,' this activity forms capitalism's human subjects, sustaining them as embodied natural beings, while also constituting them as social beings, forming their *habitus* and the socio-ethical substance [. . .] in which they move" (61). Notably, Fraser foregrounds the emotional elements of care work that contribute to subject formation and the solidification of social rules of engagement, in contrast to Arendt's focus primarily on physical sustenance through labor.

Fraser also demonstrates how late-stage capitalism draws neat boundaries between "work" that is economically sanctioned and rewarded and "labor" that is a necessary precondition for work to occur, and yet also exists outside systems of economic reward. She argues, "Wage labor could not exist in the absence of housework, child-raising, schooling, affective care and a host of other activities which help to produce new generations of workers and replenish existing ones, as well as to maintain social bonds and shared understandings" (62). Fraser is certainly not alone in arguing that care work is economically devalued or to call for compensation for labor conducted in the home (Federici), but her framework is distinct in seeing an opportunity for subversion in this labor that both undergirds and also operates outside of traditional capitalist economies.

So where does body work fall within these distinctions between labor, work, and care? One necessary precondition according to Wolkowitz is body work's relationship to compensation that specifically takes it out of home spaces and familial relational contexts and puts money at the center of the physical exchange (*Bodies*). The fact that body work is paid work is important because, as previously discussed, this is a critical gap in previous research on bodies, much of which has focused on the social construction of the body and often explicitly taken the body out of contexts of paid employment. Thus, body work frequently involves the emotional and physical labor attributed to care, especially of children and the elderly, but also maintains a focus on economically compensated care work.

Given the centrality of direct physical engagement to body work, we also might see it as more closely tied to Arendt's definitions of labor. And yet, while certain categories of body work are aligned with sustaining human life, especially a lot of healthcare work, many other types of body work are instead concerned with optimization of the embodied form (i.e., nail technicians, massage therapists, tattooists, body piercers) that is more closely tied to performance of a desired social body (Gimlin, *Body Work*). However, as Wolkowitz and Rowland have argued, this bodily optimization does not operate outside of economic relations. Instead, it is often a precursor to attaining high-paying, white-collar jobs. Wolkowitz explains, "The healthy, fit, and attractive body is not only a sign of class privilege but may be becoming increasingly central to the reproduction of professional and managerial status" ("Social Relations" 506). As one example, research has shown that having bad teeth can act as a barrier to employment (Halasa-Rappel et al.); thus, the implications of body work form a feedback loop within economic systems. Individuals must hire body workers for their own body to be socially acceptable within employment systems.

This feedback loop raises another important component in considering contemporary body work, which is that the nature of work broadly—and the body's role in labor specifically—has changed significantly in the United States over the last century. Discussing countries that are democracies with market-based economies, Wolkowitz argues that body work has replaced food and clothing production, which have been exported ("Social Relations" 499). In this new economy, "interpersonal interactions, as compared to the making of objects, is often of greater importance" (*Bodies* 1). She also points to the growth of female employment as a driving force in the increase of body work, as it transformed a significant portion of child and elder care into paid work rather than an unpaid background condition of capitalism like Fraser describes. At the same time, democratic market economies often import laborers to meet the growing need for body workers, "relying especially heavily on the migration of (often racialized) labor from poorer countries" ("Social Relations" 499). This creates the preconditions by which body work often becomes stratified along race and gender lines.

The Body

Thus far, in unpacking origins and definitions of body work, I have been homing in on "work." Shifting into a focus on the "body" draws me into material rhetoric frameworks that consider the degree to which the body is a rhetorical actant of its own. Rhetorical theorists typically approach considerations of materiality from two differing views. One approach is to view objects, environments, and bodies as sites where discourse and power are inscribed. Much like the research that Wolkowitz attributes to the "cultural turn" in sociology, attention to how materiality manifests cultural norms of gender, disability, and race has become quite popular within rhetorical studies. For example, in *Rhetorical Bodies*, the authors discuss representations of Demi Moore's pregnant body, accounts of the psychological body in mental illness memoirs, and construction of HIV-infected body through home-testing kits (Selzer and Crowley). While materiality garners attention in these discussions, agency remains with humans to inscribe materials with meaning. This scholarship also risks putting only nonnormative bodies into focus. As Chávez argues in "The Body: An Abstract and Actual Rhetorical Concept," "only when actual bodies are not white, cisgender, able-bodied, heterosexual, and male do they come into view as sites of inquiry" (246).

Meanwhile, a current shift toward materialist philosophy in the field has resulted in analyses of the persuasive capacities of materials and bodies as "actants" that exert rhetorical force and shape rhetorical situations in excess of humans and human intention. Bruno Latour introduced the language of "actants" rather than agents to describe nonhuman entities with impact. In Latour's actor-network theory, "actor-networks are assemblages of humans and nonhumans; any person, artifact, practice, or assemblage of these is considered a node in the network. [. . .] Links are made across and among these nodes in fairly unpredictable ways" (Spinuzzi 5). Thus, agency is distributed across the human and nonhuman actants that participate in the network and is accrued through increasing connections.

Building on Latour, Barad offers an agential-realist account of "intra-action," which occurs in a "causal relationship between the apparatuses of bodily production and the phenomenon produced" ("Posthumanist" 814). Toggling between a social constructionist perspective and a materialist perspective, Barad emphasizes how apparatuses are neither fully inscribed nor fully deterministic: "They are neither neutral probes of the natural world nor structures that deterministically impose some particular outcome" ("Posthumanist" 816). Thus, apparatuses create meaning in intra-action with human bodies, environments, and objects—"matter" emerges in particular moments at the interface of these nodes rather than from any of them in isolation.

As an example, Barad describes a demonstration of space quantization in quantum physics that came to matter through the smoking of a cheap cigar in the lab. The cigar is a "'nodal point,' as it were—of the working of other apparatuses, including class, nationalism, economics, and gender" (*Meeting* 167). While describing the cigar as an independent agent is misguided, Barad argues that recognizing the experiment's entanglements in gendered and class-based material practices is crucial to understanding this moment. Recent materialist rhetorical analyses in rhetoric of health and medicine similarly attend to the role of nonhuman actants, ranging from gut bacteria (Jane Bennett) to MRI dyes (Teston) to ostomies (Kessler).

Similarly, this book considers bodies as actants whose rhetorical force includes but also extends beyond human intention. Through the routinization of specific actions, bodies can learn to move of their own accord, settling into an embodied practice, or habitus, that helps them navigate professional spaces with ease (Bourdieu). These second-nature embodied practices can also be disrupted by one's own body, other people, an environment, or a rogue technology, and, as I discuss in more detail in chapter 2, disruptions provide an opportunity to reflect on and even reassess bodily action (Magelssen). Educational contexts offer a unique opportunity for studying embodied practices because they are places where students are often still consciously acquiring professional habitus. Since this habitus is unfamiliar to them, it operates at a more conscious level than it will once it becomes routinized in their workplace, making it more accessible for reflection, engagement, and even critique.

The relational dynamics that students bring to embodied encounters with patients are also instantiated within a community's genres and modes of communication. A rhetorical theory of body work recognizes the role that genres play in shaping embodied encounters and in making certain kinds of embodiment possible while foreclosing others. Bawarshi uses the example of the patient medical history form (PMHF) to argue that "the genre supports and enacts a separation between the mind and the body in treating disease, constructing the patient as an embodied object" (74). He goes on to describe how the PMHF's focus on physical symptoms also shapes the encounter between physician and patient, causing the doctor to "treat the patient as a synecdoche of his or her physical symptoms" (74). This embodied view of genre highlights how a single doctor–patient exchange participates in a network of other genres, all of which shape embodied workplace practices.

However, beyond viewing genres as informing embodied exchange, scholars have also recently been calling for a view of bodily moves themselves as genres. Or, as Weedon and Fountain argue in their analysis of teaching the engineering design process, "embodied routines and orientations can function as genres [. . .] witnessable through gesture, bodily orientation, movement, and text and tool use" (590). What does a view of bodily practices as genres bring to a theory of rhetorical body work? In line with definitions of genre more broadly, it calls us to think about embodied practices as typified rhetorical actions in response to recurrent situations that are "stabilized-for-now" (Schryer). It calls us to recognize the social emplacement of embodied actions such that they enact the values and goals of larger communities of practice but also represent individual instantiations of those values and goals. A view of bodily practice as genre highlights the relationship between environmental cues, or triggers, and our ability to leverage previous knowledge. Or, as LeMesurier argues in her discussion of somatic metaphors, "Bodily stores of affective, emotional, and physical knowledge enable us to motivate embodied movement, gesture, and posture in response to situational exigencies, but accessing this capacity requires methods of triggering this knowledge and drawing similarities between the past and current situation" ("Somatic Metaphors" 363). Part of the goal of classroom teaching, then, becomes helping students develop "learned recognitions of significance" (LeMesurier, "Mobile Bodies") to enact previously acquired "moves" at the right moment.

As LeMesurier's work suggests, central to a material approach to bodies is a recognition of their interconnectedness to environment and context. Similarly, others have conceptualized bodies as events, taking an interconnected view of mind, body, and environment: "Conceptualizing bodies as events privileges a position wherein bodies are involved in continuous connections with other bodies, rather than there being one causal point of origin as defining a body in terms of what it is and what it can do" (Coffey 7). This view of bodies as events is central in disability scholarship, which is, by its nature, attuned to mutability. As Siebers explains, disability is one identity category that all of us will experience over the course of our lifetimes. Unlike gender, race, sexuality, and class, "being human guarantees that all other identities will eventually come into contact with some form of disability identity" (5). Siebers's scholarship calls attention to the ways that both health professionals' and patients' bodies will move into and out of disabled identities over the course of their lifetimes. These experiences of disability can disrupt learned ways of moving through professional practice, the habitus that is being taught in health science classrooms. They also require attunement to each patient's unique physical experience of the world as it shifts and evolves. A theory of complex embodiment recognizes the social realities of disabling environments and attitudes but also the physical realities of experiences like chronic pain and aging (25).

Relatedly, research on disability and the body in composition and rhetoric scholarship emphasizes moment-by-moment enactment of embodied difference. For example, Kerschbaum calls for the field to move away from identity categories that treat difference as stable and "fixable" to markers of difference that emerge as individuals navigate interactions with one another and their environments. Much like Siebers's complex embodiment, "Markers of difference are always situated, negotiable, and part of individual interactions. They are also framed by and interpreted within broader sociopolitical contexts" (Kerschbaum 634). In her discussions of individuals navigating life with ostomies, Kessler notes how an overemphasis on narratives from people experiencing disability often causes material aspects like the environment, the ostomy, and the body to receive less attention (296). Her theory of rhetorical enactments incorporates language as one of many "agential cuts" that make momentary meaning of disability experiences: "Words may play a significant role in the agential cuts staged, but such cuts are only possible among all intra-active elements [. . .] such as histories, experiences, space, time, other humans, objects, and more" (315). To conceive of bodies as events is to understand them as mutable, mobile, and, in some ways, impossible to capture except in isolated snapshots. It is to shift focus toward bodies in process of becoming and in intra-action with other entities rather than static views or descriptions. It is both methodologically challenging, as I discuss below, and transformative.

Overall, in sociological theories of body work, scholars have lamented a dematerializing of the body. Wolkowitz attributes this to sociology's cultural turn, whereas Gimlin points out how "all labor that brings workers into contact with other peoples' bodies is potentially demeaning and [. . .] is typically accompanied by distancing techniques, whether via demeanor, the wearing of uniforms or exam gloves, or the allocation of less tasteful tasks to those further down the status hierarchy" ("What Is 'Body Work?'" 358). If taking the material body out of body work is a strategy for conferring status and solidifying one's position within a hierarchy, then a materialist framework for body work is even more necessary. A materialist approach can uncover the ways that unruly bodies are likely to act back against these dematerializing impulses, threatening status and neat divisions of labor along the way. A materialist approach attends to bodies and environments in moments of performing professional actions effectively and in many moments of imperfect performance as well. And for students, imperfect bodily performances are key for fueling critical reflection and visioning of a different kind of body work in the future.

Origins of Patient Sense

In line with a materialist approach to body work is the concept of patient sense, which draws on Beverly Sauer's research on the role of embodied knowledge in mining practices. Sauer's ethnographic research on risk communication in mining finds that while all three knowledge types—pit sense, engineering experience, and scientific knowledge—have embodied components, pit sense is the most directly tied to the body and a primary source of knowledge for workers in the mines. She defines pit sense "an embodied sensory knowledge derived from site-specific practice in a particular working environment" ("Embodied Knowledge" 137). For example, a change in pressure in the mine or the echoing of a falling rock might prompt miners to draw on their previous experiences and embodied knowledge to recognize that something is wrong.

A corollary to pit sense, patient sense similarly describes the embodied sensory knowledge that healthcare providers gain from physical presence alongside and in contact with the patient (Campbell, *Simulating Nursing*; Angeli and Campbell, "Intuition"). This might include physically knowing how a patient's stomach should feel when palpated or emotionally sensing that a patient is providing a misleading answer to a question. While it can be explicitly taught—for example, in conjunction with technologies like a robotic manikin—patient sense is often tacitly acquired through real-world experiences.

Given its mediating role between general anatomical knowledge and direct patient experience, patient sense can be understood as a type of phronesis, a Greek term used to describe practical wisdom. While typically associated with scientific knowledge, scholars have argued that phronesis has a moral dimension and is at least in an Aristotelian understanding an "ethico-political practice aimed toward proper judgment and action" (Smith 93). Smith argues that Heidegger uses phronesis to anchor his vision of "authentic care," a project that Teston takes up in the conclusion of *Bodies in Flux* as well, where she argues for "adding *phronesis* to the constellation of rhetorical skills necessary for contemporary medical practice" (177). For Smith, part of the way that phronesis enacts its ethics is through disruptions that provide opportunities for realignment and reflection, a return to "right desire" over technical or theoretical preoccupations (88).

This ethical view of phronesis is contrasted with another Greek rhetorical concept, mêtis, which is often translated as "cunning intelligence." Like phronesis, mêtis is connected to responsive action in the moment. According to Dolmage, however, while phronesis is "regulated by habits of character with the goal of 'truth' and wisdom [. . .] *mêtis* has the freedom to be less moral and seeks an isolated result" (11). For that reason, it is sometimes disparaged, viewed as the more deceitful counterpart to elevated phronesis, much in the way that rhetoric is contrasted with "truth" by the Greek philosophers (Kopelson 133). Dolmage compellingly argues that part of this disparagement is also tied to mêtis's affiliations with the body and with disability: "*mêtis* is denounced because it calls up bodies, and specifically the wrong bodies: the unpredictable bodies of women (like Mêtis) and of the artisan (the disabled Hephaestus)" (11).

However, given the recent interest in embodied rhetorics, scholars have found themselves drawn to mêtis specifically because of its emphasis on radical embodiment. In *Bodily Arts,* Hawhee demonstrates how ancient Greek education emphasized mêtis and subsequently recognized, "thought does not just happen within the body, it happens *as* the body" (58). Similarly, Elizabeth Britt's book *Reimagining Advocacy* examines how law students develop empathy for victims of domestic abuse in a program that includes classroom and courtroom experiences. Britt describes how across these contexts, students' empathetic learning is immersive and embodied, ultimately leading to the development of mêtis, which she describes as "embodied intelligence essential to understanding not only how to perform [practices of deference] but whether and when to do so" (83). Britt argues that mêtis is achieved through a combination of explicit instruction and opportunities for embodied practice, which enable students to identify the proper opportunities for action (123). For example, observing a student's support of a client during a trial, Britt notes how Chloe enacts client empowerment through "a physical recognition of solidarity (kneeling down beside her) and support (letting her cry)" (97).

Given phronesis's role in conversations about healthcare learning and practice (Rentmeester et al.; Rentmeester and Liebzeit; Montgomery), however, it would be misguided to position phronesis as disembodied or outside of immediate physical experience. Indeed, Teston argues for a material-feminist practice of phronesis that accounts for both bodies and "extra-human environs": "Under the rubric of *phronesis,* then, care is not a disembodied morality or a right way of acting. It is radical dwelling in and through bodies, or a way of being inclined toward the flood of tonalities that bear up and make possible that which we come to know" (178). Similarly, in connecting phronesis to healthcare providers' intuitive patient knowledge, I have argued that "phronesis allows healthcare providers, especially in novel situations, to draw on intuition and experience to navigate care—that is, they draw on their situated, embodied intelligence to act" (Campbell and Angeli 374). Ultimately, then, I connect patient sense to this embodied understanding of phronesis, recognizing that in doing so I may at times also be invoking mêtis as well. Pope-Raurk has argued that the two might be thought of as counterparts (324) or complements (327), but for me the ethical dimension of phronesis resonates as does its positioning as a praxis tied to scientific knowledge. As I discuss more in chapter 2, an embodied view of phronesis also helps to highlight the role the body can play in disruption that reorients providers toward the immediate moment and "right desire."

Given their orientation toward responsive moment-by-moment action, neither patient sense nor phronesis is easily taught through written texts. Sauer sees teaching pit sense with textbooks or in classroom contexts as an impossibility: "As they react, [miners] may draw on previous training and experience, but they do not call on texts at the moment of action to help them react" ("Embodied Knowledge" 159). Similarly, reflecting on how nurses move from novice to expert during their careers, Rentmeester and Liebzeit note that phronesis is not something that can be learned in a textbook, because "its cultivation requires thoughtful practice regarding how to navigate situations that may have aspects in common but are nevertheless ultimately unique" (3). Overall, Sauer notes that pit sense is not accounted for in any of the technical documents at the mine, in part because miners do not "record their reactions in written communication" (159). At the same time, the directions that miners receive often cue them to rely on sensory intuitions to guide their work. In interpreting a set of directions, Sauer points out the contradictory way in which "the imperative actually commands the miner to use common sense and experience to interpret sounds and visual cues to assess risk in temporally specific and site-specific conditions" (141). Thus, the document instructs miners to move beyond written instructions and leverage their pit sense during the decision-making process, a complicated imperative that creates ambiguity around who is at fault when mistakes happen.

Meanwhile, Sauer's second level of expertise, "engineering experience," accounts for how engineers gain knowledge from "physical signs or indexes embodied in objects and materials. Engineers observe and record this information as the material history of particular sites" ("Embodied Knowledge" 134). While she contrasts this with the direct sensory experience of pit sense, Sauer also highlights the intuitive work that enables engineers to move between broader scientific knowledge and descriptive local accounts. She notes that engineers must "read between the lines" and "read into" reports. She even quotes an engineer describing his process of "read[ing] into [a report] what we need to make sense out of it, trust[ing] our instincts" (151). This knowledge resembles what Fountain calls "trained vision" in his research on student learning in a cadaver lab as well.

Trained vision is a "theory of embodied rhetorical action that explains how objects, bodies, and discourses together generate a professional (in this case, medical) subjectivity that emerges in practice and is rooted in bodily activities" (Fountain 14). Given his observations of students learning anatomy in the lab, Fountain is particularly interested in the relationship between visual and tactile learning and the acquisition of a new language of anatomical parts (27). He argues that through guided dissections and class lessons, students acquire trained vision, which "plays a crucial role in structuring and generating our thoughts, perceptions, and possibilities for action, and it does so by shaping the ways our bodies respond to our environment" (194). Drawing on theorists of embodiment including Merleau-Ponty and Bourdieu, Fountain's account of trained vision recognizes a developmental trajectory by which embodied practices begin at the level of explicit instruction and intentional action. However, through repeated practice, embodied acts become "dispositional tendencies," eventually moving into a "middle ground between conscious experience and automatic, unconscious activity" (48) as students professionalize. This argument highlights the value of studying educational spaces as they become sites for embodied practices to transform from intentional to habitual, from explicit to inexpressible.

Finally, Sauer describes scientific knowledge as "physical forces, particles, materials, and interactions that are sensed or perceived as data in language, physical tracings, and inscriptions. Scientists read and interpret data to formulate knowledge that is literally invisible to the physical senses" ("Embodied Knowledge" 134). As this definition suggests, mediating technologies play a key role in the production of scientific knowledge. For example, Teston's book, *Bodies in Flux*, unpacks several of the ways that mediating technologies—from MRI visualizations to statistical formulas—create health data that becomes the basis for medical decision-making in cancer care. Overall, Teston calls for providers to "account more holistically for evidencing as a verb, a practice, or a performance—not necessarily a static and perfect object rendered expertly in a laboratory. Intra-actions between humans, nonhumans, space, matter, and time *evince*" (54). To recognize medical data as the result of performing and practicing certain kinds of ontological cuts is also to recognize that this data is not devoid of intuition and embodied patient sense.

In our research on healthcare intuition, Angeli and I unpacked a range of sensory cues that prompt provider action and intervention, arguing that embodied knowledge plays a role in the activation of all these cues (Campbell and Angeli). Our taxonomy includes internal cues that emerge through tacit knowledge and a provider's felt sense of a situation; environmental/bodily cues that are triggered by the provider's immediate situation; interrelational cues that emerge through written or verbal exchange with others; and technology cues that offer mediated information about a patient's condition (365). Mediating technologies can provide information that cues intuitive action—like the alert from the Rothman Index when a patient reaches a deterioration threshold—but we argue that practitioners still draw on their immersed patient sense, accrued through prior experience, to make sense of these cues. And the cues themselves still bear the traces of human and material performances that created them, hence the wide range of biases that we find embedded in our "neutral" scientific tools and algorithms (Noble; Benjamin).

Thus, while Sauer ultimately relegates pit sense to the domain of the miners and engineering and scientific knowledge to alternative domains of practice, our analysis of intuitive cues shows how both engineering experience and scientific knowledge still incorporate embodied and intuitive knowledge about the environment into decision-making. In a similar way, this book demonstrates how patient sense is being activated whether a provider is directly palpating a real person's abdomen or whether they are observing a patient's movements on a screen; technological mediation transforms patient sense but does not eliminate it. The providers' body and its dispositional tendencies, acquired in a variety of professional and educational contexts, are activated in both cases. For all my providers, they are consistently toggling between these different domains of knowledge, finding ways to translate their sensory knowledge for others, integrating it alongside mediated patient data, and arguing for its legitimacy and value. And as I demonstrate, physical, emotional, and discursive body work are at the heart of those negotiations.

Body Work Research in the Health Professions

While sociological research on body work has explored contexts ranging from massage therapy (Wainwright et al.) to prostitution (Wolkowitz, *Bodies*), workers in healthcare contexts have received only limited attention. The most in-depth exploration is the special issue of *Sociology of Health and Illness*, which brings together a range of essays on body work in "health and social care." As Twigg et al. describe, body work's advantage in healthcare research is precisely the ability to move between individual patient–practitioner interaction and larger societal systems: "we are better able to understand the micropolitical relations between practitioners and patients and clients, how difficult these are to alter, and how these are shaped by the wider social and economic context" (172).

Taken together, the authors in the special issue highlight the relevance of body work to health contexts, especially the physical role of the body in health providers' work and the emotional demands their jobs place upon the body. Brown et al.'s research on how gynecologists establish patient trust through a combination of linguistic speech acts and bodily acts previews this project's argument for a focus on discourse in research on body work. Meanwhile, I expand on Harris's interest in habitual action and the importance of disruption in facilitating learning in chapter 2 when I discuss the role that disruption plays in supporting empathetic learning during nursing simulations. Finally, Måseide offers important insights into the role that technologies play as virtual appendages of the practitioner's body, calling for an embodied perspective on these medical tools. However, all of these authors focus on physician or patient experience, overlooking the myriads of other health practitioners involved in bodily exchanges.

This scholarly focus on physicians and patients is a trend that I have discussed in rhetoric of health and medicine research as well ("Rhetoric of Health") and one that significantly limits the scope of our work and contributions to health research. Alternatively, this book shifts our focus to the body-work experiences of other healthcare providers—nurses, physical therapists, and tele-observers—three professions in which patient sense and physical and emotional modulation are arguably even more central than they are for physicians. As Wolkowitz has argued, it was specifically by cordoning off bodily contact that physicians gained status within healthcare hierarchies: "the construction of medicine as a professional occupation suitable for middle-class men could take place only if prolonged interaction with the patient's body was limited, and hived off, along with the tasks of 'mopping up,' to female nurses" ("Social Relations" 501).

Physical therapy and tele-observation exist ambiguously within this hierarchy of physical contact as well. Physical therapists typically have at least two years of education beyond the bachelor's, but they must work to rhetorically safeguard their expertise and status against the disempowering effects of high levels of patient physical contact. Meanwhile, tele-observation transforms a typically high-contact, low-status healthcare role into a virtual space. As such, it is still performed by vulnerable populations, specifically women of color, but the virtual context both affords new opportunities and confers new limits on these individuals. This section considers connections between theories of body work and all three professions as well as recent feminist technoscience research that takes up the relationship between technology and bodies.

Nursing

Nurses, of course, are some of the most physically interactive health providers; touch and emotional interactions with patients are at the heart of their practice. As Shakespeare explains in her literature review of nurses' body work: "They lift, they handle, they insert cannulas, they clean, they inject, they anoint, they use their hands and bodies affectively, they use and monitor complex machinery and attach it to people effectively" (47). This explanation captures both the direct body-on-body contact that characterizes much of nursing practice and the emotional work and negotiation of technologies that is central to the profession. That said, scholarship on nursing body work is limited primarily to Fisher's research on male Australian nurses' body work, which I discussed in the introduction, an article by van Dongen and Elema that discusses a "culture of body work" in nursing, and Shakespeare's literature review. Other nursing research focused on the body—such Lawler's body of work on the somology of nursing—tends to prioritize patient experience.

Van Dongen and Elema's work argues that much of body work in nursing practice operates as tacit knowledge, showing alignment with Sauer's research on pit sense: "Touch and the ways it is experienced by both [patient and nurses] belong to the silent culture of care and human interaction. By making this silent culture explicit we stand to gain more knowledge of what nursing and caring is about" (150). For my research, pedagogical contexts are unique spaces in which tacit practices are named, discussed, and even sometimes critiqued as part of students' enculturation into the profession. Meanwhile, Shakespeare's analysis focuses on how nurses' bodies are discussed in academic nursing research, and she organizes her findings around tropes of bodily engagement including backbreaking work, tender touch, and multisensory engagement (seeing, hearing, etc.). She ends this discussion with a call for more research on how people "do" nursing, noting that much of the research in her study was based on retroactive interviewing rather than in situ observation: "one real investigative possibility lies in exploring methodic practices of which bodywork actually consists. *How do people do nursing*, how do people use their bodies in a competent way and how do they use their bodies to show that they are competent?" (54), a call I take up, although my interests extend far beyond demonstrations of competence.

Physical Therapy

Like the scholarship of nursing, there are a handful of studies considering body work in physical therapy practice or adjacent fields. Many of these studies focus on the relationship between body work and professionalism or expertise, specifically considering how the embodied practices of providers work to reaffirm or potentially undermine their professional status. For example, Norris and Wainwright's article on learning professional touch in physiotherapy, which involved observations and focus groups with year one and year two physiotherapy students across two terms, argues for a longitudinal process of professional development in students' use and understanding of touch. This process begins with hyper-self-awareness and a reliance on peer feedback; progresses toward more comfort and a focus on interaction through touch; and shifts again as students move into clinical practice and come to see touch's role in establishing relationships with their patients and communicating care.

Norris and Wainwright note that many of students' concerns throughout this progression—like self-control and breaching of social and physical barriers—are tied to concerns about professionalism (95). The authors also argue that physiotherapy education still overemphasizes physical and biological knowledge without sufficiently attending to the social dynamics of bodywork encounters. The program's encouragement of students "smack[ing] right through" normal social barriers to get comfortable with all kinds of touch does not sufficiently account for "the concerns of individual dignity and negotiated acceptability emphasized and expected later" (97). Thus, they support curriculum revisions that center touch as a "complex social encounter" (99).

Wainwright's prior scholarship has taken up similar concerns about professionalism and body work but with a focus on young mothers in body-training courses that teach massage and reflexology. Wainwright et al. show how paradoxically, while the classroom-salon emphasizes the women's "natural" predilection for the work as an extension of their maternal identity, instructors also encourage students to tone down their femininity to desexualize the environment and highlight scientific expertise (84). Technical knowledge and scientific concepts as well as physical measures like wearing uniforms professionalize participants but also distance them from the body, patient sense, and "perceived skills developed through everyday lived practices" (84). In a similar way, George's study of body work and personal training argues that trainers accrue status outside of traditional communities as "expert service workers" that must negotiate the line between catering to clients' needs and maintaining professionalism, "attempting to draw their authority from their specialized training" (115). The physical therapy students in my study were often quick to draw boundaries between themselves and personal trainers, given their many more years of formal training. Still, they shared some of the challenges described by George in navigating care that necessitates that they act responsively to client needs, relying on moment-to-moment patient sense to inform decisions while also enacting professionalism through references to scientific expertise.

Tele-Observation

Of course, the concerns raised in body-work research on both nursing and physiotherapy about negotiating professional and personal boundaries and reifying expertise are even more complicated in virtual environments. As professions that have historically relied on physical patient interactions shift into virtual spaces, the nature of body work is transformed, at times into information work (Sandelowski 67). Sandelowski explains how virtual contexts challenge the importance of "presence," which has often been identified as a core contribution in professions like nursing and physical therapy: "the new virtual geography [. . .] calls into question how essential bodily presence is to being there and to patients' feeling that their nurse is there for them" (63).

At the same time, this removed bodily presence has advantages for experienced practitioners who may confront physical and emotional burnout from the ongoing demands of body work in healthcare. Van den Broek's interviews with twenty tele-nurses demonstrated that "remote-nursing technologies presented nurses with opportunities to 'rub off' or significantly reduce the physical and psychological damage they faced in ward-nursing roles" (906). Her study tracks themes of the "perforated body" from interviewees who innumerate the small, consistent physical and emotional wounds of floor work, as well as the "regenerative possibilities" of telework, even if it comes at the expense of career advancement. Tele-observers present an interesting contrast, since those I interviewed represented a much more diverse range of backgrounds and experiences in healthcare.

And yet, a posthuman approach to virtual healthcare would have us recognize that these divisions between information work and body work are false binaries that reify a Cartesian dualism. As Sandelowski envisions it, in a truly transformed nursing practice, "These nurses will be able to conceive of the body work of washing, toileting, and turning patients as information encounters, and ultrasonography, genetic counseling, and the entry of data into the computerized medical record as embodied encounters" (67). This call for embodying virtuality and making patient sense visible even in its mediated forms is reminiscent of feminist technoscience work that posits the cyborg body as a future vision for feminist work, blending technological and embodied knowledge rather than rejecting either approach (Haraway).

Calling practitioners toward a cyborg ontology in healthcare, Lapum et al. argue that "person-centered practice can be actualized in the contextualized, embodied and relational spaces of technology" (276). A virtual intensive care unit certainly offers an opportunity to observe this actualization in real time, as novice practitioners negotiate relational care and leverage embodied patient sense in virtual spaces. And as Twigg et al. argue, the advantage of a body work framework for healthcare is its attention to the micropolitics of care (172). At play in these micropolitics of care are a wide range of power-based hierarchies that are both particular to the healthcare context and tied to body-work frameworks more broadly.

Body Work and Hierarchies of Power

As the previous sections suggest, research on body work is always inextricably linked to considerations of gender, race, and class—the distribution of power across bodies. Sociological theories of body work emphasize how it is devalued within social and institutional systems and frequently gendered as "women's work." These connections are diverse and wide-reaching—from the rise of women in the workforce leading to a corresponding rising demand for paid body labor (nannies, housekeepers, etc.) to the racial implications of reserving the "dirtiest" body work for the most marginalized populations like migrant women (Wolkowitz, "Social Relations"). Alongside the devaluation of body work and its allocation to vulnerable individuals is its persistent invisibility. As a society, we often look past the people who keep our spaces and bodies clean and healthy.

Rowland's book *Zoetropes* demonstrates this tendency to overlook those performing bodily labor. Her book attends to the discursive practices that constitute humanhood at sites including the American Gut Project, the National Memorial for the Unborn, and elite fitness centers. However, in her chapter on vital biocitizenship at the gym, she reflects on how she did not consider interviewing the janitorial staff until much later in her project when a reviewer suggested it. The staff, a team of Latinx women, was responsible for the pristine look of the gym, but their body work frequently happened at the margins of gym participants' awareness: "Those women wiped clumps of hair from shower drains, gathered soiled towels from the floor, restocked supplies, emptied waste bins, and cleaned toilets—in other words, they performed the repetitive, physically demanding, and poorly paid labor of maintenance" (121). I experienced a similar phenomenon in my work in the virtual intensive care unit (VICU) that I describe in chapter 4. My initial observations in the VICU were focused on the nursing team who was responsible for monitoring algorithms and patient participation in various wellness programs. It was not until after I had completed a summer of observations and had some distance from the project that I realized that I was really interested in the experiences of the tele-observers on the other side of the room.

This section begins to unpack some of the convolutions between body work and power distribution across bodies, with a focus on race, class, and gender. While I separate these three components in my discussion here, the separation is artificial. Many, if not most, body workers are multiply marginalized, and their workplace oppression intersects with cultural patterns of oppression in society writ large. Because of these knotted overlaps and convergences, it feels overly simplistic to just point out that women of color occupy so many of the least-valued and lowest-paid body-work positions. And yet, this is also how the intersections between body work and systems of power are made most apparent.

When I go about my day-to-day life in the city of Milwaukee, I see the predominance of female immigrants from Asian countries working as nail technicians in a nail salon, of Latinx women taking care of my daughter at her daycare, of Black women drawing blood and giving shots in our doctor's office (Campbell, "Not Just Doctors"). I can compare this with the more highly paid body workers in my life who are still women but are all white—the hairdressers at my high-end salon, my barre instructors, the doctor and nurses at our pediatrician's office. These are patterns and there are, of course, exceptions—but one of the clear advantages of the body-work framework is that it highlights the connections between bodily work and systemic oppression.

In part, the invisibility of body work is tied to historical legacies of racism. Different racialized bodies are expected to move differently—in different spaces, taking on different roles, and with different physical movements and levels of visibility. These expectations emerge in everyday interactions and performances as well as through media representations. For example, in her essay "Winking at Excess," LeMesurier analyzes how Childish Gambino repeatedly moves between two of these social expectations for Black male kinesiology—that of talented entertainer and that of threatening Black man. She argues that Gambino's oscillation between rhythmic movements that draw on African traditions of dance and hyperviolence forces the audience to also move between different affective attachments to his movements: "When he dances, we are comfortable. The moment he takes hold of a gun, we cringe reflexively" (148). His dancing also demonstrates the constant demand for the Black male body to be in motion, "via a kinesthetics of entertainment that is marked by excessive, spectacular skill" (140). While Gambino demonstrates expectations for Black male bodies in public spaces, these racialized kinesiologies inform our expectations for individual embodiments in all kinds of professional contexts.

For example, in chapters 2 and 3 I discuss instances of student laughter during a nursing simulation and in the physical technologies lab. Laughter is, on the one hand, a physical response to experiences of awkwardness for students as they navigate uncomfortable conversations. It can also support in-group bonding and identification (Magelssen). But laughter is also tied to power, and learning to control one's laughter is part of the emotional modulation that students are acquiring in their classrooms. Who is allowed to laugh and when is connected to the racialized and gendered kinesiologies that LeMesurier describes as well.

To better understand how these racialized expectations come to be, one must look beyond a single national context and instead recognize body work as tied to the international circulation of labor. Hochschild has used the term "global care chains" to describe the commodification of care and love (the "new gold") as they move from poor countries to affluent societies in the form of household care providers (*Commercialization*). Examining the experiences of migrant domestic workers in Hong Kong, for example, Yam notes how their home countries often promote these roles because of the economic resources that are brought back home in the form of remittances, even with the knowledge that foreign countries have exploitive policies in place (121).

In fact, training programs in countries like the Philippines specifically educate domestic workers in affective management to endure exploitative working relationships, especially since the participating women are often overqualified for caregiving roles. Lagman's interviews with Filipina caregivers identifies two specific affective strategies—disaffection and discernment—that contribute to their ability to navigate intimate, familial relationships with their employers. Disaffection, much like Hochschild's concept of emotional management, involves channeling strong affective responses to appear unmoved to employers. Meanwhile, discernment involves introspection about the origins of emotions, their history, and their relationship to others' feelings (12). Lagman argues that affective management strategies like these constitute higher-order rhetorical navigation for participants in her study than the skills that are traditionally considered complex, like language learning and communication

(3). She also notes how workers in more "skilled" positions, like nursing, education, and IT, still frequently emphasize the embodied and emotional aspects as their work, again breaking down assumptions about what constitutes higher-order work (4).

Hochschild's framework of global care chains, which was constructed specifically to describe nannies working in domestic homes, has been critiqued for its inability to account for transnational circulation of highly skilled labor, especially in the health professions (Wolkowitz, *Bodies* 160). However, as Lagman's research demonstrates and this project seeks to highlight, body work is no less relevant for skilled providers in these roles, even if their work does not take place in the bedrooms and kitchens of their employers. Meanwhile, considering body work raises new challenges in these international contexts for a wide range of providers because bodies move and act differently across cultural divides. For example, Harris's research on body work of overseas doctors working in Australian hospitals notes how they must undergo processes of sensory adjustment to adapt their patient sense in a new cultural context for care: "a process of situated, embodied, sensory learning, continually oscillating between their past and the present" (309). These sensory adjustments often occur through moments of mismatch between doctors' tacit patient sense and the current situation, which disrupts habitual action and subsequently prompts bodily adjustments (310). Bloom-Pojar makes a similar argument about the embodied communication practices of US health professionals providing care in the Dominican Republic, arguing that their "translanguaging" practices went far beyond linguistic translation to include gesture, empathy, and a range of strategies for reading bodies. Notably, however, in the Dominican context, the provider has professional power and state power, a reversal of the power dynamics often present in global care chains.

Overall, differentiating between professional roles by categorizing higher- or lower-order skills quickly proves to be problematic, especially when one tries to sort these skills based on cognitive versus embodied components. Indeed, Lagman's observation that "skilled professionals" in her study described their work as "embodied and emotional, not solely cognitive" (4) comes off as self-evident on the one hand. Of course, nurses and teachers, especially those navigating new cultural contexts abroad, would find that work to be emotional and embodied. But on the other hand, her statement speaks to larger assumptions about how body work corresponds to class—the assumption that high-skilled, high-paying, white-collar work operates in the realm of the "mind" while low-skilled, low-paying, blue-collar work occurs at the level of the body.

Mike Rose's *The Mind at Work* specifically takes up these classist divisions to demonstrate the complexity of embodied labor in fields like hairdressing, plumbing, and carpentry. In line with Lagman's argument that embodied skills can, in fact, be "higher order," Rose calls for a greater valuing of working-class bodily intelligence. At the same time, he recognizes how many blue-collar and service jobs are institutionally deskilled, routinized, and regulated in ways that "limit, often severely, the various forms of meaning one might gain from [them]" (xlviii).

Along with classist assumptions about what constitutes knowledge work come gendered assumptions about the appropriate realms of body work for women and men. In working-class communities, jobs that entail physical labor like mining (Sauer; Ivinson and Renold), welding (Mackiewicz), and car repair (Cushman) are reified through their associations with masculinity. In their study of body work and working-class boys in ex-mining communities in Wales, Ivinson and Renold note how their participants "opt to retain the masculine identities which value making and doing above writing, because they associate these practices with the kinds of jobs they imagine being able to secure in the future" (277). Importantly, the authors view the physical literacies of boys in Wales as born of intergenerational systems of bodily knowledge "that enabled young men and boys to be brought up to endure long shifts of physically demanding labour in dangerous conditions underground" (289). Meanwhile, these physical literacies are often incompatible with the body-work practices that are expected in school settings, especially during crucial literacy performances like exams. Thus, Ivinson and Renold argue that part of addressing working-class boys' underperformance in school is better accounting for body work that has deep community and social value, as well as intergenerational legacy.

Masculinity is not just valued in working-class work environments, but its valuing does transform in white-collar workspaces often into an emphasis on objectivity and rational argument and the disparagement of emotional or embodied engagement, which is frequently feminized. As Acker explains, "masculinity always seems to symbolize self-respect for men at the bottom and power for men at the top, confirming for both their gender's superiority" (145). Again, distance from bodily engagement confers professional status in these workplaces, which poses a particular problem for health providers whose practices are firmly grounded in touch and embodied knowledge (Wolkowitz, *Bodies*).

For example, in Wainwright et al.'s study on mothers learning body techniques, the authors argue that these courses take an ambiguous position on the role that gender and motherhood play in providing "innate" bodily knowledge for participants. The instructors "shift between gendered notions of the innate and developed, as well as the academically taught. Skills in relation to bodies and emotions are perceived as natural and intuitive at the same time as technical and in need of learning" (81). Appeals to technical knowledge act in part to defeminize knowledge and desexualize the embodied context of the environment, even while they are often "justified primarily on the grounds of health and safety and professionalization" (84). Mulla makes a similar observation about female forensic nurses working with rape victims, arguing that they produce a "clinical competence that is professional while not appearing overly empathetic or caring" (15). In part to distance themselves from the victims, the nurses appropriate the removed, masculine persona that aligns with law enforcement.

Of course, when women do speak and perform from a place of embodied knowledge, their communication can offer a powerful counterdiscourse to masculine ideologies that dominate professional contexts. As Knoblauch argues, "an embodied rhetoric born from embodied knowledge can disrupt what is often assumed to be an academic or professional mastery [. . .] and can rattle loose the privileged white masculinist discourse" (62). In a chapter about clinical simulations, I have shown how both the overt and implicit pedagogy of simulations teaches students lessons about how to perform their gender and orient to others (Campbell, "Simulating Gender"). At times, these lessons resist a hospital culture of objectivity and distance and position the nurse as an advocate for the whole patient's embodied experiences. This book builds on that research and other scholarship on body work in healthcare to consider how gendered, racialized, and class-based performances intersect with physical and emotional maintenance in the education of healthcare professionals. I also argue that a rhetorical approach to body work can foreground attention to hierarchies of power in bodily exchange and offer pathways for more equitable practices.

Rhetorical Field Methods

While writing scholars have recently focused on questions related to students' work experiences (e.g., Brittenham; Lu and Horner), and rhetorical scholars have taken up explorations of embodied knowledge (e.g., Hawhee, *Bodily Arts*; LeMesurier, "Mobile Bodies"), attention to the body/work nexus has been limited in both fields. For example, the edited collection *Bodies of Knowledge*, which explores embodied rhetorics in a range of private and public contexts, only features one chapter that addresses workplace embodied practices. In her chapter on Tammy Duckworth, Osorio unpacks how Duckworth's physical presence on the Senate floor as a woman of color in a wheelchair with her infant daughter on her lap challenges social expectations surrounding motherhood, work, governance, and disability (143).

Meanwhile, feminist rhetorical scholarship has called for more attentiveness to gender as it intersects with professional discourse and action. The book *Women at Work* argues that there has been an overemphasis in feminist scholarship on women's civic participation, which can also lead to a focus on white, upper-middle-class women (Gold and Enoch). Hallenbeck and Smith suggest that "'work' has been both ever-present in [feminist rhetorical] scholarship and simultaneously, somewhat tacit, invisible—under-theorized as a discrete area of study" (201). Similarly, Frost has introduced a methodology of "apparent feminism" designed to "make apparent the urgent and sometimes hidden exigencies for feminist critique of contemporary technical rhetorics" (5). She argues that masculinist values like efficiency in the contemporary workplace contexts are often tacit and normalized, necessitating a critical feminist approach.

Overall, there is a pressing need for more research that articulates intersections between professional practice, rhetoric, and embodiment especially in the health professions. Calls for such work have been ongoing, from Haas and Witte's discussion of gesture in engineering writing, which argued that we talk a lot about writing/embodiment but rarely study "the real-time, material, corporeal action[s]" that constitute writing (417), to Clayson's call for a "distributed writing" approach to professional composing that accounts for embodied practices. Along similar lines, Twigg et al. lament the predominance of interviews in sociological research on body work: "Empirical research is dominated by interviews, in which the experiences of workers and patients are translated into words, with the inevitable bias towards abstraction and bleaching out of the corporeal. There is [a] paucity of observational work" (175). And yet, it is not surprising that both fields have struggled to acquire observational data from active worksites; ethnographic fieldwork comes with many barriers including access to sites and extensive time investment. However, for projects that are committed to unpacking and analyzing embodied practices, fieldwork, coupled with video recording when possible, is irreplaceable.

In "Staging Fieldwork/Performing Human Rights," Madison explains how ethnographic fieldwork immerses the researcher's body in their research context: "Something happens differently when your body must move and adjust to the rhythms, structures, rules, dangers, joys, and secrets of a unique location. Ethnography is as much, or more, about bodily attention—performing in and against a circumscribed space—as it is about what is told to you in an interview" (401). For Madison, fieldwork allows the researcher access to physical aspects ("rhythms, structures"), emotional aspects ("dangers, joys"), and intangibles ("rules," "secrets") of a given space. This access to a wide range of tangible and intangible aspects of a rhetorical context is well aligned with an expanding definition of rhetoric that aims to better account for embodiment and materiality and resonates with several components of a rhetorical body-work framework.

As scholarship in both rhetoric and writing studies demonstrates, fieldwork enables scholars to recognize and value nontextual and nonverbal aspects of communication from gesture to interactions with objects to affective inclinations. It also supports better accounts of audience engagement and response (Middleton et al.). For projects like mine that are invested in understanding communication as embodied, affective, and environmentally situated, I considered this access to be imperative. Thus, in all three of these projects I adopted an "ethnographic perspective" that combined in situ observations with interviews and document collection. I detail the scope of my fieldwork at each site in the analysis chapters, but across projects I valued frequent presence in students' and providers' learning environments. This presence allowed access to the physical and emotional experience of interactions in the moment and enabled me to better understand each of these unique rhetorical contexts. As previously mentioned, the "My Body on the Scene" sections in each chapter identify my own positionality and experience during a specific moment of the research process.

Rhetorical field methods exist on a spectrum between those that aim for detailed descriptive accounts of practice and those that take a critical rhetoric orientation interested in unpacking systems of oppression and power and accessing marginalized voices (Middleton et al. 390). While rich and useful, the descriptions of local practice have the potential to elide issues of power and difference between human actants (Jung). In my research, it was important to recognize educational spaces as places where power relations are being both explicitly taught and tacitly acquired. As Britt points out, "rhetorical education is always about power relations—about who can participate and in what forms" (4). Thus, I was committed to observing how lessons in body work were also concerned with teaching students to orient to powerful and marginalized positions. As new nurses, how were they learning to orient toward a disabled patient? As future physical therapists, what lessons were they learning about stroke victims? How did tele-observers' learning about empathy in CNA training translate to virtual observations?

In my efforts to enact a methodology that was attentive to the circulation of power and difference at my research sites while still aligning myself with their pedagogical missions, I found feminist rhetorical theory to be instructive. A key principle from Royster and Kirsch is "critical imagination," referring to a new way of engaging in analysis and critique that is open to inventive possibilities and grounded in the experiences of those being studied: "we gain a deeper understanding by going repeatedly not to our assumptions and expectations but to the women—to their writing, their work, and their worlds" (20). Their focus on patience and careful attention to local experiences resonates with Krista Ratcliffe's theory of rhetorical listening and her articulation of "standing under" discourses of another to experience immersion prior to critique. Ratcliffe advocates, "Consciously standing under discourses that surround us and others while consciously acknowledging our particular—and very fluid—standpoints. Standing under discourses means letting discourses wash over, through, and around us and then letting them lie there to inform our politics and ethics" (28). These authors challenge scholars not to approach people and texts with preconceived agendas and instead to bracket assumptions and be immersed in the conversation.

Extending Ratcliffe's emphasis on recognizing our own standpoints, Middleton et al. express concern that rhetorical fieldwork has given little attention to the body of the critic: "Rhetorical scholars could learn much from our performance colleagues by more rigorously considering our own bodies and how they interact with the interpretive frameworks and situations we enter when critiquing lived rhetorical experience" (396). The authors note that self-reflexivity is often granted a paragraph in the methods sections of these analyses rather than a sustained position throughout the critique. Taken together, these authors emphasize a necessary toggling between immersion in the discourses of others and awareness of our embodied position and perspective in that immersion.

In many ways, my position as an outsider at these research sites supported this consistent toggling during my fieldwork. During clinical simulations, for example, the coordinator would readily remind students each time she reintroduced me that I was "not a nurse" and, therefore, "was not judging them." Meanwhile, my status outside of the health professions was clearly marked by my lack of medical clothing—students in simulations and tele-observers in the VICU wore scrubs. In interviews, I noticed that students would occasionally make the same translational moves for me that they made for patients during a lab. Thus, I sought to remain attentive both to the range of interactions, perspectives, and emotions circulating at my research site and to my embodied experience of the situation to fully leverage the affordances of an ethnographic methodology. Throughout this research I oriented toward my research sites in an immersive way where I could "stand under" the circulating discourses and remain aware of my own perceptions and interactions.

At the same time, I incorporated video recordings into my analysis when possible to disrupt and redirect my initial impressions of situations and to challenge myself once again to move away from simplistic critiques. As I mention in the introduction, I had video recordings available for the first two case studies—clinical nursing simulations and the physical therapy lab. Access to video recordings enabled me to account for relationships between verbal comments and gestures, positioning and movement around the classroom space, and interactions with classroom objects. Similarly, some of the research on professional writing has begun to take advantage of video recording for greater access to the materiality of professional communication. For example, Haas and Witte's article uses video recordings to consider the role of gesture in a collaboration between city officials and engineers to revise a visual/textual document.

Meanwhile, video recordings allowed me to account for student actions in more detailed and precise ways than with field notes alone, by transcribing and coding data for material and embodied practice. I saw video recordings, along with student interviews, as sources for disrupting and redirecting my assumptions about exchanges. In this way, they worked in tandem with a feminist analytic orientation that aimed for immersion in the research site and attentive engagement with the discourses that circulated there, not fixating on critique but still attending to lessons in power relations that were both explicitly taught and tacitly acquired.

Applying a Rhetorical Body-Work Framework

This chapter has traversed a diverse range of academic scholarship in establishing a theoretical groundwork for rhetorical body work and the concept of patient sense. I began with the definition of rhetorical body work as paid physical, emotional, or discursive labor performed at the material or technological interface of worker–client bodies. Important to this definition is the notion of body work as paid work (Arendt; Fraser). This focus addresses a critical gap in previous research on bodies, which frequently emphasizes care work in the home or civic participation (Wolkowitz, "Social Relations"; Gold and Enoch; Hallenbeck and Smith). I also introduced feminist materialist approaches to both the body and technology, which, rather than analyzing representations of the body, instead attend to the body as a rhetorical actant that participates alongside other actants in meaningful events (Barad; Spinuzzi; Teston). In conversation with disability studies (Siebers; Kerschbaum), this perspective recognizes all bodies (providers' and patients') as mutable and "stabilized-for-now" (Schryer). Disruptions to learned ways of moving and intra-acting can emerge at any moment from one's own body, the patient's body, the technology, or the environment. Indeed, even in my own research practices I sought to "disrupt" my own critical habitus to encounter my participants and their experiences authentically.

I also drew on Sauer's theory of "pit sense" to elaborate the concept *patient sense*, embodied sensory knowledge that healthcare providers gain from physical presence alongside and in contact with the patient. I align patient sense with the Greek rhetorical concept of phronesis—practical wisdom—which recent scholars have recognized can be just as deeply embodied as its corollary concept mêtis (Teston; Campbell and Angeli) but also carries an ethical commitment toward authentic care (Smith). In conversation with Sauer, I argue that patient sense is activated whether a provider is directly palpating a real person's abdomen or observing a patient's movements on a screen; technological mediation transforms patient sense but does not eliminate it. Discourse is also an active part of learning patient sense for providers—they must find ways to translate their sensory knowledge for others and to argue for its legitimacy and value alongside mediated data that comes from patient charts or technologies.

Finally, I reviewed existing research on body work in nursing, physical therapy, and telemedicine as well as the relationship between rhetorical body work and distributions of power across bodies. I demonstrated that research on body work is always inextricably linked to considerations of gender, race, and class. The most vulnerable populations are often the ones performing the lowest-status body work (Wolkowitz, *Bodies*; Hochschild, *Commercialization*) and are also often "invisible" to researchers and the public (Rowland). Societal expectations for embodied practices are tied to racist and classist assumptions about how bodies are expected to move (Ivinson and Renold; LeMesurier, "Winking"). These assumptions emerge in part due to global chains of economic exploitation that circulate bodies for profit, at the same time disciplining those bodies into practices of physical and emotional modulation (Lagman; Yam; Hochschild, *Commercialization*).

Having established a clear theoretical basis for this project, the remainder of the book applies a rhetorical body-work framework and the concept of patient sense across three related healthcare contexts—clinical nursing simulations, a physical therapy lab, and a virtual intensive care unit. While my process for researching these three sites was somewhat serendipitous, as I describe in the field context sections of each chapter, they are united by a shared focus on embodied healthcare practices and technological tools. They are also all pedagogical contexts, which I have highlighted throughout this chapter are spaces where habitual embodied actions are made explicit and denormalized. The virtual intensive care unit is somewhat of an exception in this regard, but my interviews with tele-observers focused on the diverse range of formalized and ad hoc experiences that buoyed their current work. Thus, even though I was not observing tele-observers in the process of learning embodied practices, I did hear many accounts about tele-observers' learning experiences. Given that their education was informal and varied greatly between participants, a retrospective approach was the only way to access it.

While these three sites share an embodied, technological, and pedagogical perspective, they also each offer unique insights into a theory of rhetorical body work. The first chapter on clinical nursing simulation begins from the premise that empathetic patient relationships are central to nursing practice and identity. Thus, it explores the role that robotic manikins can and cannot play in the acquisition of empathetic body work, demonstrating the ongoing necessity for teaching empathy in technologically mediated contexts. The second chapter recognizes the precarious disciplinary positioning of "touch professions" like physical therapy, caused in part by their proximity to the body and reliance on patient sense. It explores how boundary-work aimed at maintaining disciplinary prestige is enacted physically and verbally through body work and the gendered implications of those enactments. Finally, the third chapter explores the diverse training and experience of tele-workers, demonstrating how their unique mediated patient sense and body work draws on both their professional histories and their emplacement in the shared space of the virtual intensive care unit. In doing so, it argues for greater attention to body-work experiences and training that occur outside of traditional four-year education and that leverage intuitive knowledge gained in a range of extracurricular and professional contexts.

Across all three chapters, I recognize and value the ways that new health technologies are transforming professional body work in healthcare, requiring new kinds of physical, emotional, and discursive practice. These shifts are truly cataclysmic, restructuring access to providers, distribution of resources, and hierarchical relationships between professions. And yet, a rhetorical body-work framework also keeps bodies in focus with emphasis on the very human elements of empathy, expertise, and intuition. All three elements draw on a wide range of physical (palpating an abdomen); environmental (hearing a falling instrument); and technological (noticing increased beeping on a heart-rate monitor) cues. And all three are based in the body—impossible to disentangle from its moment-by-moment interactions with the world and others.

CHAPTER 2

A Feeling for the Robot
Embodying Empathy in Nursing Simulations

In 2010 the University of Minnesota Medical School announced that it would be moving away from hiring paid actors for second-year students to practice pelvic exams and that students would be working exclusively with a manikin-based model with sensors that can provide feedback on student touch (Bannow). A female graduate student wrote an editorial in response to the article arguing against the standardization of bodies in health education and aligning this with a larger cultural critique about representations of the female body: "In an era where women's bodies are continually objectified and encouraged to look more and more like a Barbie Doll, it is truly disturbing to see our bodies being literally replaced with plastic dolls in the training of the professionals who will care for our bodies" (Kesti). And indeed, the vision Kesti provides of a line of future doctors learning a highly personal and invasive exam on a lineup of identical, peach-colored plastic torsos is a disturbing one. It is also not one that matches my own experiences with clinical simulations when I spent a year following a group of junior-year nurses through their simulation training in a clinical performance lab.

Instead, the students in my study were deeply immersed and actively engaged in a wide range of patient interventions and care—from palpating a swollen ankle, to asking about the patient's relationship to his dad, to deciding how to document their care on a large whiteboard. In teams of three, the nursing students moved rapidly around a fully stocked mock hospital room, where the robotic manikin was only one feature among many that was meant to cue their burgeoning patient sense and enrich their understanding of nurses' body work. Indeed, many of their cues came from the simulation coordinator, Maura, as she spoke through a microphone connected to the manikin's mouth, thereby giving the patient a voice and an ability to respond to care.

A perfect representation of a future patient? Absolutely not. But also, not an experience that was entirely detached from the physical or emotional needs of a real patient either.

When asked what distinguishes them as health professionals, most nurses will cite empathy as a key component, developed out of extended patient contact, both physical and emotional (Campbell and Miller; Bas-Sarmiento et al.). Nurses often spend more time on the clock with patients than any other health professional at the hospital (Butler et al.). Thus, they are expected to have a more holistic view of patient experience that they can bring to conversations, document in charts, and carry forward into patient care. For many student nurses, this opportunity to deeply know their patients and to act as patient advocates within a system that can often be dehumanizing is precisely what draws them to the field. They anticipate a career of emotional and embodied patient exchange, in which their consistent physical presence alongside their patients—their patient sense—is critical to their knowledge and contributions within an interprofessional health landscape. To say that rhetorical body work is at the core of the nursing profession, then, is an understatement. This expectation of responsive and patient-centered practice, however, is perhaps why the idea that health professionals are learning patient care on high-tech robots can be an affront to the public's expectation for what health training should be.

Kesti's critique is in line with prior gender studies research on patient simulation that I discuss in the introduction (Johnson; Sundén). These critiques seem born of two related concerns. First, outsiders express fear that the patient manikin cannot physically represent a "real patient" or the tactile experience of patient interaction. This is, at its core, a concern about how practitioners' physical patient sense might be muddled through acquisition on a "plastic doll." Second, there is a concern about emotional patient sense—that future nurses and doctors will not practice emotionally connecting with their patients and empathizing with their experiences if their learning takes place on a manikin. Both concerns make the mistake of viewing patient manikins as static objects and critiquing their inability to replicate a real person physically and emotionally. However, materialist feminist scholarship calls our attention to the necessity of focusing on simulators as "apparatuses in action" (Johnson; Sundén) that through intra-action (Barad) shape future practitioners' patient sense. Thus, this chapter asks: If embodied and emotional patient connection and understanding is at the center of nursing practice, what role do patient simulations that center robotic manikins play in acquiring that empathetic body work? Or put more simply, can robots teach patient-centered care?

To answer this question, this chapter first overviews connections between simulation and empathy, arguing that disruption is central to how simulations move from being focused only on knowledge acquisition toward fostering critical perspectives and meta-awareness. This is important because nursing simulations are disruptive precisely because of their inability to perfectly replicate the physical and emotional cues that facilitate patient sense on the job. Next, I discuss the history of experiential learning in healthcare training and the structure of simulations at Northwest University. As I analyze simulations through the lens of rhetorical body work, I discuss how the patient preparation sheet is designed to discursively cue physical and emotional patient care and then move into discussions of the physical and emotional learning that students experience during simulations. In both cases, while instructors put a good deal of effort into ensuring the fidelity of the simulation environment, its imperfections disrupt student care.

Importantly, these disruptions contribute to students' lessons in body work because they destabilize habitual action and prompt reflection, approximating many of the ambiguities that students will experience on the job. The chapter concludes by considering the risks of acquiring physical and emotional body work in simulation contexts through discussion of a troublesome example. Here, the physical and emotional cues in the simulation designed to approximate the patient sense of a hospital room intra-act to culminate in a problematic moment of cultural insensitivity. This raises questions about the limitations of pedagogies of empathy and points to the need for strategies that can help students to grapple with difference without devolving into stereotyping or assumptions.

Embodied Empathy and Simulation

Empathy as Body Work

Empathy is often understood as the practice of embodying the emotions and physical experiences of another. When that other is a paying consumer—a client, a customer, or a patient—empathy constitutes body work, physical and emotional labor performed as part of economic exchange. Blankenship's research also positions empathy as rhetorical by tying it to invention, discourse, and narrative. She defines rhetorical empathy as "a choice and habit of mind that invents and invites discourse by deep listening and its resulting emotion, characterized by narratives based on personal experience" (5).

Notable here is her reference to "deep listening," a concept that draws on Arlie Hochschild's work on surface versus deep acting (*Managed Heart*).

When surface acting, a worker performs emotions that they are not actually experiencing, like smiling even if they are unhappy. When deep acting, a worker consciously changes their emotional state to feel the emotion they are performing, like empathizing with a difficult patient by relying on stereotypes about that patient's demographic group (Lindquist 197). For example, Gimlin describes how a provider might "consciously reorder elderly people as sweet, innocent, and vulnerable [. . .] to overcome their feelings of disgust" ("What Is Body Work?" 362–63). One can already see how the notion of deep acting quickly complicates the view that empathy is always a desirable, or moral, stance for a provider. In simulations, where instructors may not share the identities of the patients they are performing, these issues are complicated further, as the final example in this chapter highlights.

Despite the fraught nature of deep acting, most scholars are adamant that empathy cannot be practiced without a willingness to fully take on and embody the experiences of another. Many acknowledge that this goal is unachievable, and we will ultimately be faced with what Leake calls "a recognition of unknowability" (i.e., awareness that there will always be psychic and physical distance between oneself and another). However, Lindquist argues that the path to taking on an empathetic habitus must involve deep acting: "When you deep act [. . .] you work, through acts of will and imagination, to open yourself up to the possibility that you might persuade yourself that the emotions you are presenting as real. You risk becoming the thing you are performing. Deep acting is, paradoxically, the process of exerting control in order to relinquish control" (197). Deep acting, then, also helps counter the power imbalances that can arise when someone in a dominant position attempts to take on the perspectives of the marginalized, one of the primary risks of empathy. In deep acting, the empathizer creates the possibility of change for themselves by truly experiencing the other's world.

The notion of deep acting also calls into question pedagogies of empathy that are primarily focused on encountering narratives of another's experience, like those that are widespread in medical humanities programs. While these programs provide access to patients' perspectives in the form of illness narratives, they offer students little in the way of experiencing empathetic practice in communication with a patient (Campbell, "Rhetoric of Health"). Without that praxis, "personal narratives—whether real or fictional—can serve an individualizing function that obscures social, political, and economic licenses and constraints" (Kulbaga 510). In addition, without experiencing the embodied enactment of empathetic practice, empathy is likely to remain on the level of surface acting and risks repeating the erasure of the marginalized through overidentification. Overall, rhetorical scholars tend to highlight how empathetic practice is not only cognitive or emotional but also embodied. To feel what others feel, to see what others see—such vivid imagining can be understood through the Greek rhetorical concept *energeia*, which Roundtree describes as "bringing before our senses the potency and virtue of the actual thing" (85). Simulations work to center the body in empathetic learning, then, in ways that arguably cannot be achieved through literature or narrative alone.

One way that empathy is centered during simulations is that the instructor or clinic coordinator provides a voice for the patient and can prompt empathetic engagement through their responses to student care. Whether she was asking students to translate medical jargon, expressing anxiety, or reacting with surprise when students did not warn her before removing a garment, Maura provided regular reminders that their patients were not just bodies. My interviewees all noted that these interactions during the simulations did more to elicit empathy than activities where they were asked to embody the perspectives of their patient through physical modifications.

For example, junior-year nursing students in my study participated in an activity geared toward helping them appreciate the physical experiences of aging. They wore heavy body suits, distorted glasses, and uncomfortable shoes, and then had to try to do everyday activities like walk around and eat pudding. My interviewees had universally negative reactions to these simulations, however, much in line with disability studies critiques of activities that ask students to simulate disability. As Siebers explains, "Disability simulations of this kind fail because they place students in a one-time position of disability, before knowledge about disability is acquired, usually resulting in emotions of loss, shock, and pity at how dreadful it is to be disabled" (28). In appropriating the experience of disability without the subsequent embodied knowledge of how to navigate the world with that disability, then, these simulations foster pity rather than empathy.

The Importance of Disruption

Scholarship on simulation emphasizes the distinction between simulations of reification, which reinforce the status quo, and those of invocation, which imagine possibilities for change or innovation (Magelssen). Crocco describes this second category as "critical simulations," explaining: "If successful, the critical simulation will produce cognitive dissonance between one's pre-conceived notions about a domain and the new experiences generated by the simulation; this opens up a space for critical reflection and analysis." Crocco's emphasis on "defamiliarizing the domain" and producing "cognitive dissonance" highlights the important role that critical simulations can play in challenging participants' worldviews. However, Crocco's emphasis is cognitive without recognizing how defamiliarization can happen through embodied disruptions and meta-awareness can be physically triggered (LeMesurier, "Mobile Bodies").

Certainly, clinical simulations like those in nursing are invested in assimilating nursing students into a disciplinary community with particular values, views, and goals. However, they are designed not just for skill acquisition but also to support the development of problem-solving, communication, and embodied learning. In the process, they prompt enactment and reflection on power relationships in clinical settings and promote a view of nurses as patient advocates and forces for change in a dehumanizing medical world. This advocacy is not simply discursive but embodied and enacted in each move that nursing students make while practicing patient care.

One of the key distinctions between assimilation-oriented simulations and those that create the capacity for change is the presence of disruptions. I use the word *disruption* to describe actions that disturb, redirect, or overturn the existing simulation scenario and force students to act reflectively and responsively. Disruptions are closely tied to patient sense because they emerge when a physical or emotional experience does not match our engrained expectations, whether it is a gut feeling that something is not right (Campbell and Angeli) or the sound of falling rocks (Sauer, "Embodied Knowledge"). Being able to trust this knowledge and appropriately respond to a disruption becomes part of the embodied practices of a professional. In clinical nursing simulations, the manikin's disruptions are brought about by its imperfect representations of a human, while the instructor's disruptions are often strategically introduced to prompt emotional response. In both cases, disruptions provide opportunities for students to reflect on how they will modify their care for different kinds of bodies, supporting an awareness of variation and flexibility with interventions.

In theorizing phronesis—practical wisdom—Smith has also pointed to the importance of disruption. Phronesis disrupts habitual ways of knowing and doing that emerge out of a fixation with technical knowledge and a kind of preplanned, optimized existence. Phronesis, through its radical immediacy and responsiveness to the world, resists technological complacency. According to Smith, "Such disrupting would seek to destabilize the stability of the spaces, *doxa*, habits, practices, norms, signs, narratives, concepts, subject-positions, and social institutions that are the very 'ground' of communal life" (100). Connecting these arguments about disruption and technological complacency to patient care, the authors of "A Cyborg Ontology in Health Care" describe the important role of disruption for healthcare practice:

> The inherent danger is that a mere technological, habitual way of being does not permit us to be open to the embodied and contextualized experiences of patients. A disruption of the habitual in terms of logics, embodiment, and routines can move nurses and other healthcare professionals to a conscious integration of patient centered practice into the technological care environments. (Lapum et al. 286)

The authors see disruption as a means for calling healthcare workers back to embodied and situated patient care in situations where technology has routinized practice. Their emphasis on "conscious integration" points to the value of disruption for fostering meta-awareness of one's actions as well. When one's expectations and plan of action do not fit reality, this provides an opportunity to reassess and even question actions that have been routinized.

What becomes apparent in the interactions between students and manikins in the excerpts I examine here is the many ways in which the machine disrupts and redirects students' practice—necessitating that they negotiate difficult conversations about ambiguity and recognize the wide range of variation within "normal" human bodies. Manikins are designed specifically for fidelity of intra-action, so that students' sensual experiences anticipate those they will encounter with a real patient. In her research on medical simulation, Prentice describes how the physical experiences of surgery must be "parsed, calculated, incorporated into the computer's programming" to design effective simulators (83). This closely resembles Sauer's discussion of designing robots that can approximate pit sense as well (139). Even still, the manikin body is disruptive during students' care—too heavy, too resistant, too male (Campbell, "Simulating Gender").

In fact, to return to the scholarship on empathy, scholars argue that disruption provides the means for a productive distancing that can help foster critical empathy. DeStigter describes critical empathy as "the process of establishing informed and affective connections with other human beings [. . .] while always remembering that such connections are complicated by sociohistorical forces that hinder the equitable, just relationships that we presumably seek" (240). Others also point to the importance of emphasizing both similarity and difference in critical empathetic practice, noting points of identification and recognition without collapsing important structural differences between individuals (Ratcliffe 99). If empathetic learning and practice is always a balance between embodied immersion and critical distancing, disruption in simulations becomes a means for productive redirection that can foster this reflective distance. As we move into considering how body work is taught in the context of clinical nursing simulations, then, disruption is a central component in understanding student embodiment.

A Brief History of Experiential Learning in the Health Professions

Perhaps more so than for other professions, educating future health practitioners necessitates visual and physical encounters with the body. Foucault believed that clinical training represented a unique instance of the "appropriation of discourse" because rather than learning language practices, students were being trained to appropriate a clinical gaze that took the symptom as symbolic. In *The Birth of the Clinic,* Foucault argues that the shift to apprenticeship models of doctor training at the end of the eighteenth century was also marked by this visual shift in pedagogical practice. Even prior to that, dissection halls in early fourteenth-century Italy used cadaver-based anatomy lessons to transfer what Fountain calls "trained vision" from expert practitioners to novices (5). Starting in the late Middle Ages, "The practices of dissection, demonstration, and observation communicate this authoritative knowledge [of the body] to those who seek to reveal the body's supposed secrets. For centuries, the activities of cutting, presenting, and viewing human bodies have dominated medical education" (Fountain 7). Anatomy labs still play a role in medical education today, though there has been reduced emphasis on dissection in favor of practice on models of body parts with sensors, like the pelvic models described in the opening of this chapter (Prentice 35).

Meanwhile, professionalization in nursing began in the United States after the Civil War, when more than three thousand women served as nurses providing care for the sick and wounded. Many of those women would go on to establish nurse training schools, the first of which opened in 1872 (Egenes 6–10). In these hospital-based apprenticeship programs, nurses would provide two to three years of free care in exchange for clinical lectures. Thus, the foundation of US nursing education was experiential, with learning happening on the clinic floor. The apprentice system received critique, however, and after a multiyear examination of nursing education concluding in 1923, the Rockefeller Foundation published a report recommending that schools of nursing needed to focus on education rather than patients and should develop more rigorous educational standards (Egenes 19). Still, the growth of baccalaureate and graduate programs in nursing was slow even into the 1960s, with most nurses participating in hospital-based certificate programs. The 1964 Nurse Training Act increased federal funding for nursing programs and brought about the growth of graduate nursing programs and the spread of baccalaureate nursing education (Egenes 21). Today, nurses in the United States can practice with a diploma in nursing from a three-year certificate program, but these programs are rapidly decreasing, and most nurses receive either an associate's or bachelor's degree (Egenes 23).

Coinciding with the rise of baccalaureate nursing school was the rise in experiential teaching with patient actors for health practitioners. In 1963 a neurologist at the University of Southern California (USC), Dr. Howard S. Barrows, began to teach third-year medical students using actors that had been trained to exhibit various conditions—what he referred to as "programmed patients" (Rosen 161). Collaborating with Stephen Abrahamson, the director of research in medical education at USC, Barrows recruited a model from the art department, Rose McWilliams, to play a paraplegic patient (Patty Duggar) with multiple sclerosis for a group of third-year neurology clerks (Press 314). Much like the editorial responding to the use of pelvic models, the media sensationalized McWilliams's role in medical education, describing her as a sexual object for the predominantly male medical students (Press 314). Ultimately, Barrows faced ongoing pushback at USC and relocated to establish a medical school at McMaster University, where he continued to develop experiential medical education (Press 315).

Barrows frequently traveled to other medical schools to spread his knowledge about programmed patients and demonstrate the Patty Duggar case. On one such visit, Hilliard Jason at Michigan State University's Office of Medical Research became inspired to design "difficult patient" cases for his own students. Press marks this as a critical moment in the development of standardized patients, as the attention shifted from a focus on symptoms toward patient personalities. She states, "Whereas Barrows developed cases based on neurological disorders, Jason focused on the characters of the patients themselves. In other words, medical students were no longer simply evaluating patients' bodies for illness but assessing their characters as well" (316). Ultimately, in her rhetorical history of standardized patienthood, Press connects Jason's approach to a larger pedagogical practice that trained students "to read patients for patterns that would directly impact their credibility of character and narrative" (316).

In her narrative about her experiences working as a standardized patient, "Empathy Exams," Leslie Jamison demonstrates the way these clues play out for her specific patient who suffers from conversion disorder, sublimating grief about her brother's death in the form of seizures. Jamison reflects on how the medical students' success in her scenario depends on empathetic engagement:

> Empathy is always perched precariously between gift and invasion. [. . .] Humility means [the students] ask questions, and questions mean they get answers, and answers mean they get points on the checklist: a point for finding out my mother takes Wellbutrin, a point for getting me to admit I've spent the last two years cutting myself, a point for finding out my father died in a grain elevator when I was two. (5)

Jamison's essay is both a critique of the assessment of empathy in these standardized patient encounters and a philosophical dive into the nature of empathy: the thin line that divides it from pity, from appropriation, from apathy.

At the same time as Barrows was spreading the word of experiential learning in medical education, his collaborator at USC, Stephen Abrahamson, was also at work with physician Judson Denson on SimOne, a human patient anesthesia simulator. In collaboration with Aerojet General Corporation, the two designed a prototype that looks in many ways like contemporary patient manikins; SimOne could breathe, show a pulse, and respond to drugs (Rosen 161). Despite early prototyping, however, it would take much longer for this technology to become widely accessible for the training of healthcare providers. Laerdal introduced their first "SimMan" manikin in 2000, which was followed quickly by other manikin manufacturers who began including software, training scenarios, and monitor interfaces to encourage schools to choose their product (Rosen 162).

The simulations that were the subject of my study blend elements from both early dissection and anatomy labs that focused on anatomical learning and standardized patient encounters. I focused on simulations that were "sequential decision-making classroom events" and used high-tech robotic manikins that respond to care both physically and verbally (Hertel and Millis) (see figure 1 on the next page). These computerized manikins are programmed to mimic breath sounds and pulses, and their vital signs respond to student intervention. For example, their temperature might rise to indicate that an infection is worsening, or their pulse might quicken in response to a medication students administered. The manikins can sweat and cry, have nasal and oral secretions and reactive pupils, and make breath, bowel, and heart sounds—all controlled by a dashboard outside of the simulation room. Shots can be injected into a pad in their arms, though oral and rectal medications are verbally described by students. Most importantly, the manikins "speak" through a microphone in their mouths also connected to the coordinator, so students can converse with the manikin and hear its reaction to their care. I

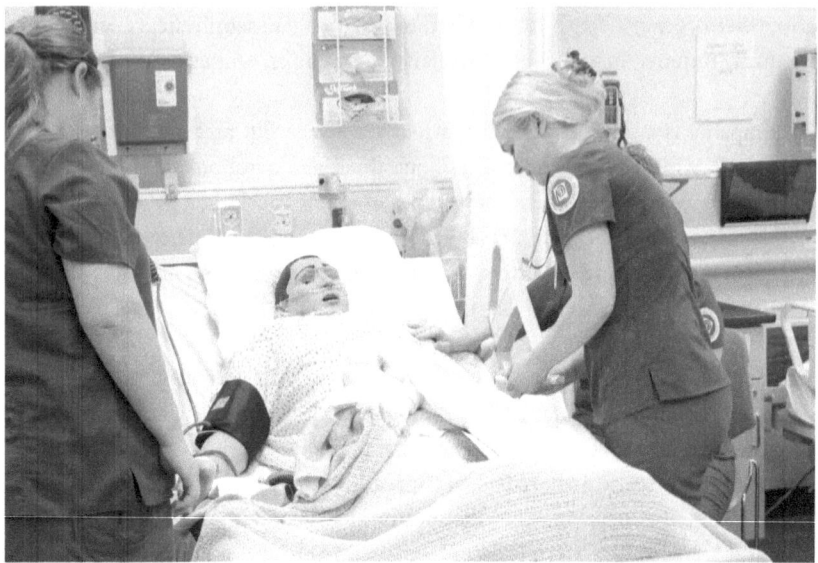

FIGURE 1. Several nursing students provide care for a male robotic patient at the Charlotte Tate Haq Nursing Lab. (CC-by-2.0) Ser Amantio di Nicolao for Piedmont Virginia Community College. Acquired via Wikimedia Commons. No changes made.

did not examine some of the more skill-based learning that students did in the simulation lab, like when they practiced inserting a catheter on a plastic pelvis using proper sterile technique.

I argue that the clinical simulations in this study provide explicit lessons in body work for students, offering opportunities to rehearse the embodied practices of their future professions in ways that are both closely aligned with future care but also importantly distinct from it. These simulations also provide physical experiences with patient sense—a swollen leg, an infected wound. Since patient sense is tied specifically to the physical and sensory experiences of the clinic, textual encounters in a classroom cannot create that knowledge (Sauer, "Embodied Knowledge" 159). Simulations work to bridge this gap between classroom and real world by approximating the physical and emotional cues that providers will experience on the job.

Field Context

The Clinical Simulation Lab

My research on clinical nursing simulations took place during the 2014–15 academic year at Northwest University, a liberal arts school in a Pacific

Northwest city with a student body of approximately 7,500. I found my way to this lab through a series of referrals and conversations, first discovering that my graduate institution conducted simulations in an ad hoc way that would not be a good fit for longitudinal research. By contrast, Northwest University had a much smaller cohort of students and a systematic approach to simulation; when I met with their director of simulation and she asked me who my theorist was, sharing that her dissertation relied heavily on Heidegger, I knew we would be a good fit.[1]

The simulation coordinator at Northwest University was Maura, and she was my main point of contact for much of the research. Maura's full-time job was designing and organizing materials for the simulations, orienting students to the process, and running simulations for all nursing students at the university. She had worked for many years as a nurse and clinical instructor but had been working full-time in the simulation lab for the past several years. This gave her a deep physical sense for clinical nursing practice as well as the particularities of embodied experiences in the simulation context. A large part of Maura's job was physical, organizing medical supplies in the suites, "dressing up" the manikin with a wig or bra to change genders, and controlling the manikin's physical reactions to patient care on a dashboard. At the same time, however, her responses to student questions were critical in shaping the direction of a simulation and had a significant impact on the body-work lessons that students learned, as I discuss in more detail below.

At Northwest University, I followed a group of about eighty third-year undergraduate nursing students over the course of the year, observing all three of their simulation events in the Clinical Performance Lab (CPL). The CPL occupies 20,000 square feet on the fourth floor of an urban medical center and is used by undergraduate and graduate nursing students. The CPL includes five low-tech (called "low fidelity") simulators used for teaching basic assessment and skills (adult and infant CPR, lung sounds, central lines), seven mid-fidelity manikins used for simple simulations and basic assessment (lung sounds, heart sounds), and two high-fidelity simulation suites with manikins that can run over ninety different scenarios (the neonatal intensive care unit and the adult intensive care unit).

---

1. The clinical director's question about my theoretical framework helped me to recognize that she would be interested in a humanistic project on simulation. Overall, I have found nursing to be very receptive to humanistic orientations, with many in the field using familiar theorists (Foucault, Heidegger) and methodologies (discourse analysis, narrative analysis). While by no means a Heidegger expert, I knew that he was a theorist of phenomenology, a branch of philosophy that is interested in everyday practice and experience. Heidegger is a popular theorist among health practitioners because he spent a decade delivering an annual two-week seminar to health professionals about philosophical theories of medical practice (Rentmeester et al.).

During simulations, I sat with Maura and the students' clinical instructor in the simulation control room, which is positioned between the two simulation suites. While Maura was in the lab full-time, the clinical instructor supervised students both at their hospital sites and during their simulations and stayed with the same group of students all semester. When I began my study, Maura gave me the choice of sitting in a corner of the simulation suite or sitting with her and the instructor in the control room. This was a difficult decision, as being in closer proximity to students as they participated in the simulation would have given me more direct access to the energy in the room and a better sense of how they were experiencing the narrative. However, I also felt strongly that my presence in the room would be a source of stress and disruption.

In the control room, the large window is one-sided, so that instructors are not visible to the students in the room. Meanwhile, the computer on the main desk controls all the patient simulator's vital signs, and a microphone is connected to the simulator's voice box. Another microphone speaks from the sky to students, playing the role of "eye in the sky" and responding to their questions about the simulation and its limitations (e.g.: Can I draw blood on the manikin?). From the control room, Maura can manage the cameras in the suites, zooming in and out to focus student attention on different aspects of the simulation for those observing in the classroom.

The two simulation suites each include a patient simulator—Joe/Josie in the adult suite and Hal in the OB/pediatric suite. During her brief tour of the room, Maura reminds students of the location of all the supplies they will need for care (gloves, a sharps container for used needles, oxygen, catheters, blood drawn IVs, etc.). There is also a computer in each room with a medication database available so students can look up specifics about any medication. Next to the computer is a phone that connects into the control room. Students verbalize who they are calling and Maura or the clinical instructor fields the call. The "medication room" is a cart on the other side of the room. There is also a large whiteboard in each room that the students use to collaboratively chart the patient's information. Before the simulation, Maura gave the whole group time to reacquaint themselves with the simulator and agree upon a template for charting.

Overview of Simulations at Northwest University

In clinical nursing simulations, students are immersed in a particular narrative set up by the simulation coordinator that gives them an opportunity to take on the roles of nurses providing care to a patient. At Northwest University, baccalaureate nursing students begin working with the simulators during the last quarter of their sophomore year of study. They start on the low-tech manikins, practicing communication, basic drug administration, and bed changing. By the end of their junior year, they are practicing in both the high-tech adult and infant simulation suites. Meanwhile, they are also enrolled in coursework and beginning their clinical placements at local hospitals.

In the simulations I observed, three groups of two to three students each took turns caring for the patient for approximately twenty minutes while the patient's condition worsened. During their turn, students practiced conversations with one another and with the patient, engaged in critical thinking to problem solve, identified possible causes of complications, and decided on interventions. They also had physical interactions with the simulation environment and the manikin—applying sanitizer, putting on gloves, adjusting the patient's dressing gown, checking wounds, and so forth. While one group provided care, the other two sat in a nearby classroom watching a video stream of the simulation on a screen. After each group's turn, the students, clinical instructor, and simulation coordinator reconvened in the classroom to debrief the simulation sequence, talking about what went well and where there was room for improvement.

I observed a total of three simulations over the course of the academic year, all based on patients and scenarios created by the educational designer, CAE Healthcare. The first involved an elderly female patient, Eliana Ruiz, who was diabetic and experiencing complications with wound care after a recent leg operation. The second was with a young male patient, Jason Lee, who was recovering after a leg surgery prompted by a recent car accident. And the third was caring for a male infant, Eric Joslin, with a respiratory infection. Despite the age and gender differences between Eliana and Jason, the same white male robotic manikin was used for both simulations, with some minor modifications.

While the simulation room and event are designed to create a cliniclike experience, there are anomalies to the space that influence student care. For example, the experience of sim stupor is a physical/emotional experience that is specific to the simulation context; its panoptic design causes students to experience that added sensation of being watched. Meanwhile, *simisms* was a term used to describe behaviors caused by the physical cues in the simulation room; for example, students forgetting to change their gloves because patient fluids are not visible.

I was very fortunate that video recording was already part of the simulation lab's practices, since students who were not participating in the simulation would watch it livestreamed from a room next door. I collected recordings and observed all the junior-year class's simulations for the year—a geriatric simulation in the fall; intensive care simulation in the winter; and pediatric simulation in the spring—for a total of approximately ninety hours of observation. By taking field notes during observations, I was able to strategically return to my video recordings to rewatch critical moments. I also conducted semistructured interviews with five focal students over the year, once at the beginning of the study and once after each simulation, during which they would reflect with me on key moments and interactions from their simulation (see appendix 1). Finally, I collected patient documentation they had written based on a simulation for our last conversation, and we discussed their writing strategies and approach.

My Body on the Scene: "Sim Stupor"

One of the dynamics that Maura alerted me to early on in my observations was "sim stupor." She described how sometimes students "go a little brain dead" once they enter the simulation room. Their focus becomes narrow and task-oriented so that they start to miss the big picture of the simulation. Maura explained: "It's like the camera lens in a movie zooms in and limits your field of view so that you can't see outside of that one area of focus. You walk in and it's a little surreal, there's lots of lights, lots of sounds." Maura intentionally sent the students' clinical instructors into the simulation room to give patient hand-offs so that they could experience the stupor for themselves.

I had my own experience with sim stupor late on a Thursday afternoon when the rest of the performance lab staff had already headed home. Needing an extra person to complicate students' care for a pediatric patient, Maura asks me to be a disruptive visitor. I was supposed to play the part of a distant relative to the other toddler in the room, bringing him strawberries to snack on, which his whiteboard indicated he is allergic to. However, as I came into the simulation room and introduced myself to the students, I misspoke and told them that I was the toddler's mom rather than his aunt/cousin. During debrief, one of the students mentioned that she did not question the snack I was bringing because she assumed that the child's mother would know what he could and could not eat. Thus, even my small error redirected the action of the simulation in an important way.

In addition, I was supposed to try to pick up Eric Joslin, the students' patient, who my character did not have any relation to. Several times, I made my way to the side of the bed, reached in and touched the baby, asking if he was doing okay. The students were aware of my presence and kept trying to redirect me and move me away from the baby. However, I never worked up the courage to pick Eric up. After my brief stint in the simulation room, I spent the rest of the simulation thinking about how I should have been more assertive about picking up the baby and rethinking all the ways I could have said or done it better. This affirmed for me the physical and emotional reality of sim stupor, and the importance that Maura gave to making sure that instructors could recognize it and be sympathetic about its impacts on student performance.

Discursively Cuing Body Work: The Patient Preparation Sheet

Prior to their simulation, students in my study received a preparation sheet from their clinical instructor with information about the simulated patient they would be caring for. While it was a seemingly minor document, my observations of simulations and interviews with students found that the patient preparation sheet did discursive work by providing physical and emotional cues that might not be present in the simulation space itself. Thus, these documents prompted certain kinds of body work from students. The preparation sheet offered a simulation-specific version of patient sense, at times requiring students to read between the lines or interpret facial expressions in a photo to gain patient knowledge that would not be spelled out explicitly in a chart. While this experience does not replicate how patient sense will manifest for practitioners on the job, it does require them to be intuitive and attentive in similar ways, recognizing that a patient's needs will rarely be spelled out without additional interpretive work.

The patient preparation sheets are designed by the educational design company CAE Healthcare. They include a photograph of the patient as well as their age, weight, and social/family history. They also include a brief paragraph entitled "Situation," which details their patient's medical history and context; a list of "Initial Orders"; a list of simulation objectives; and a list of preparation questions. The summary of the patient's "situation" in the simulation preparation sheet often mimicked information that would be provided during a nurse hand-off at the hospital. For example, the preparation sheet for Jason Lee, the patient in the intensive care simulation, specifies that

> Jason Lee is a 22-year-old male being transferred to the General Surgery/ Trauma Unit from SICU. He was admitted via the ED yesterday after he sustained bilateral compound femur fractures following a MVC in which he rolled his truck. On admission to the trauma center, his blood alcohol concentration

(BAC) was 0.12 mg/dL. His urine and toxicology screen was negative for all other drugs. After immediate treatment in the ED, he was taken to surgery for an ORIF of both femurs. Due to prolonged anaesthesia and EBL of 800 mL in surgery, he was transferred to the SICU for overnight observation. He is now stable and ready for transfer.

Here, students are given information about pre-existing conditions and allergies, past medical history, and context on where the patient has been in the hospital and what treatments have been given. Notably, the preparation sheets also include an image of the patient that genders and racializes them. Thus, the patient profiles discursively cue students to attend to difference in their physical and emotional body work in a context where the manikin is frequently unchanged.

Because students are given the chart prior to the simulation, they have an opportunity to look up information about conditions and risks and to ask follow-up questions of their clinical instructor during the preclinical conversation. Some students also tried to decipher clues about a patient's unique background and needs and used the sheet to shape their interactions with the patient. In this way, the preparation sheet cued emotional body work and specifically patient empathy even prior to interactions.

For example, under geriatric patient Eliana's social history, it read, "Lives alone and has no insurance." I had a conversation with focal student, Liz, about how she prepared herself to communicate during this first high-fidelity simulation her junior year. She came back to that note in the preparation sheet and described how it had really informed her interactions with Eliana:

> So in the chart [. . .] it said that the patient was very concerned about having to take care of herself at home and I thought that that was sort of a big red flag. Obviously, no one wants to be in the hospital. Like if someone's hurt they don't want to be there. But if there's going to be a problem when they leave the hospital, what does that mean for the patient? There's probably going to be a lot of worries. And I wanted to try to talk to the patient and ease those worries and figure out what could be the cause of it. Hopefully see if we can come to an understanding in how we can make it better for her. So that was my thought process going into it, I don't know if it conveyed fully in trying to talk to her.

In fact, Liz's thought process did come through in her conversations with Eliana, particularly when she approached her during the end of the simulation, lightly touching her arm and asking, "Ms. Ruiz, can we chat for a minute?"

She began by referencing the preparation sheet, "I saw on your chart that you live alone. Do you have any relatives that live nearby?" As the conversation unfolded, Liz found that Eliana did have a daughter in town but only talked to her infrequently because "she's awfully busy though and I try really hard not to be a burden." Liz was able to encourage her to call her daughter and let her know about her fall the accident and, in doing so, ensured more support when Eliana did leave the hospital.

Liz's reflection and the conversation that ensued demonstrate the way that a simple note in the patient preparation sheet stood in for patient sense she might have gained interacting with Eliana and informed how she oriented to Eliana in their exchange. Rather than acting as a static "assignment sheet," the preparation sheet shaped the simulation exchange, cluing students into important details and potential problems, but also setting the groundwork for conversations with the patient that could help address their social and emotional needs in responsive ways.

Similarly, the image of the patient on the preparation sheet also individualizes the patient when the manikin cannot be individualized, even when wigs, glasses, earrings, brassieres, and so forth were added to the white male model. Comparing the images provided for Eliana Ruiz and Jason Lee helps illuminate how these images provide initial cues for students on the background and unique needs of the patient. Eliana's dress is visible in an upper-body photograph of her, which shows a thick gray sweater, a crimson scarf, and a black hat. Her dress is conservative and somewhat traditional, cluing students to the fact that modesty should be prioritized during her care. Neither Eliana's dress nor her skin color call attention to the Latina heritage suggested by her name. Her description lists her ethnicity as "Hispanic" but specifies that she can speak English with the nurse. Eliana's facial features are relaxed and she is smiling slightly. This prepares students for a friendly and cooperative patient interaction.

In contrast to Eliana's composed and kind image, Jason Lee's image emphasizes his immaturity, and skepticism, as well as his racial identity. He is pictured as an Asian male wearing a gray T-shirt with medium-length dark, tousled hair that suggests youth. Most notably, Jason's expression is one of exaggerated skepticism. His right eyebrow is comically arched upward, while his left eyebrow remains turned down and his left eye slightly squinted. His mouth is in a neutral position. While this image offers the possibility that Jason could be a combative patient, I found that he was played more as curious and overwhelmed by the simulation coordinator, Maura. He certainly asked a lot of questions about his treatment and care but did not challenge the nurses' actions or decisions throughout the simulation.

While a seemingly small detail in the patient record, the images play a distinctive role by personalizing patients for the simulation. In interviews, the students mentioned repeatedly that their ability to communicate with the patient effectively relied on their seeing the patient not as a manikin but as a person. As focal student Michelle explained, "It's always weird talking to a piece of plastic because ultimately that's all he is. I kind of just take to heart the 'treat the manikin like you would treat a patient' thing, so I kind of just try to ignore the fact that it's not an actual human." Here, she references Maura's advice during room orientation to "make it real" and treat both the simulation space and the manikin as if it were a real hospital context.

Focal student Ryan similarly emphasizes the necessity of not seeing the patient as manikin: "I just talked naturally. You know I didn't have to think about how I would I talk to a manikin because it wasn't a manikin to me." Many of the focal students mentioned that having Maura's voice come from the manikin was a key component in helping them to humanize their patient. Providing an image of the patient on the preparation sheet also links individualized characteristics and even a particular clothing style to a name in ways that support this individualization.

Liz's discussion demonstrates how the patient preparation sheet could lead to empathetic reflection on a patient's unique positioning that could ultimately translate into responsive patient care. At the same time, there was also the possibility that this demographic information could make students feel more distanced from a patient. For example, focal student Kira reflected on how her close proximity in age to Jason made it easier to connect with him in conversations while she struggled more to connect with elderly patient Eliana:

> It definitely went better this time because I thought of [Jason] more as a person. I feel bad because I did think of [Eliana] as a person but there's kind of a disconnect too with age. [. . .] I feel like with [Eliana] last year there's a certain amount of respect that you give to your elders and there's a generation gap. It was easier to talk to [Jason] and pretend he was a normal person because he was our age, so it could be like a Facebook conversation or like a phone call or something.

This is an important moment because it demonstrates the risks involved with empathetic alignments that are built on shared experience. Empathy built on a premise of sameness quickly meets its limits and will ultimately privilege those that are more similar to the providers who offer them care.

Despite the potential risks of empathy built on shared experience, instructors I observed often leaned into the premise that demographic similarities would be an effective means to build patient connection. For example, Maura would regularly have Jason ask a male nurse questions about the catheter. During focal student Ryan's shift, Jason (played by Maura through a microphone) called Ryan over, saying:

> JASON: It's kind of embarrassing. How long do I have to have that tube in my penis? [...]
> RYAN: So you're on day one right now. So you'll have it until tomorrow.
> JASON: Okay yeah it's—I didn't want to ask the other nurses.
> RYAN: I totally understand.

Later on, when Ryan informed Jason that he was going to clean the catheter, Jason responded, "I'm glad it's you." Overall, Ryan discussed these exchanges positively during our interview: "He was like, 'Oh I'm glad that it's you because I don't want that other nurse to look at me' and then, it made sense. Before now I never understood why it would be an issue that I was a male but now I understand when a male's more comfortable with me, that fell into line, which was cool." Thus, for Ryan the exchange with Jason represented a rare instance where he felt his gendered perspective was uniquely useful. He describes clarity from the exchange about how his gender will sometimes be an asset. Of course, not every male patient will feel comfortable with another man talking about or examining his genitals. In fact, Fisher's study found that male nurses often navigated a lot of discomfort from male patients about touching their genitals.

At the same time, while Jason's attitude toward male caregivers helped Ryan feel valued in his simulation, identification also comes with risks of "erasure and alienation" (Morris 164). Indeed, one of my women focal students, Liz, described feeling distanced from Jason: "the patient was definitely more comfortable with a male figure just because he was male, so didn't want us to impose as much." If one assumes that patient connection is created through shared experiences, when nurses cannot easily identify with patient experience—because of age, gender, race, class, or disability—this can create a barrier to relationship-building. This is why feminist scholarship is calling for new ways of imagining how connections might be built between individuals to account for and value their different experiences (Ratcliffe; Royster and Kirsch).

From the perspective of body work, it is notable how discursive cuing in the form of the preparation sheet and the instructors' voicing of the patient set the groundwork for lessons in emotional body work for students. In this way, seemingly small image choices or prompts stood in for on-the-job patient sense to help students gain an understanding for how they will build emotional connections with patients. Overall, these moments should not be underestimated, and designers as well as instructors must be strategic about what lessons they want to teach about encountering difference through this discursive cuing.

Physical Body Work: "Hands on, Ears on, Eyes on the Patient"

During their orientation to the simulation room, coordinator Maura reminds students that even though the patient's vital signs are visible on a telemetry machine,[2] they should not rely on this information. This is an interesting instance of pushback on technological cuing that prioritizes patient sense acquired through physical touch. Maura emphasizes that "you should have hands on, ears on, eyes on the patient at all times." What this means in practice is that the simulator, specifically, and the simulation environment, more broadly, have an active rhetorical role in the simulation and that they persuade in a range of physical, visual, and auditory ways. While the patient manikin is designed to approximate patient sense on the job, it is also disruptive in its imperfect performances. This does not undermine the value of simulations but does mean that students are regularly toggling between cues that appropriately prompt their physical body work and engagement and those that require reflective negotiation and response.

Overall, the clinical simulation environments were designed with embodied learning in mind. Maura thought strategically about how to create the right feel for each scenario to facilitate the acquisition of patient sense. For example, Karen, who was a clinical instructor who worked with Maura on all the infant simulations, described their aim to create a chaotic, challenging environment for students that would best represent the experience of a pediatric ward: "We want them to feel the stimulus, the increase in sound and movement, of having a lot of people in the room." Karen's emphasis on feeling highlights how she and Maura were quite intentional about the experiential impact they wanted simulations to have on students. They would use this larger vision for the "feel" of a simulation to make decisions about what

---

2. Telemetry machines are used in most hospitals to track a patient's condition by aggregating data from sensors on the body such as blood pressure, heart rate, temperature, etc. If you can picture a patient heartbeat flatlining in a movie or television scene, that is typically shown on a telemetry machine. The data on simulation telemetry machines was controlled by the same computer system that controlled the robotic manikin.

kinds of disruptions to introduce. For example, with the goal of "feel[ing] the stimulus," multiple visitors were introduced during the pediatric simulation including distressed parents, siblings, neighboring patients, parents of the neighboring patients, and so forth.

Last-Minute Disruptions

However, Maura was not always able to anticipate every disruption she wanted to introduce at the beginning of a simulation, which led to some mismatches between the prepared objects and the scenario as it unfolded. In the following excerpt from the second round of simulations, student nurses Sean and Stephanie are part of the third shift caring for Jason Lee, the twenty-two-year-old patient who has just had surgery on both of his femurs after a car accident. The students are anticipating that a blood clot that the previous shift located in Jason's left calf through palpation is going to move to his lungs.[3] Before this final group's turn, Maura has decided to add an allergic reaction to a medication as an additional complication—something she has not prepared the manikin for physically. The following conversation unfolds as Sean and Stephanie physically negotiate Jason's care and the unexpected allergic reaction.

> SEAN: [*Rubbing anti-bacterial gel on his hands and addressing Jason.*] Yeah, Stephanie will double-check the medications. We're going to try and get that taken care of for you right away. I understand what it feels like to be itchy.
> JASON: It's really annoying, it's just . . .
> SEAN: And you said it's all over, no particular area? Not maybe just your leg? [*Pulls latex gloves from the box nearby the head of the bed and walks around the bed to Jason's right-hand side.*]
> JASON: No, I mean I just feel that it's like my stomach and my neck.
> SEAN: [*Putting on exam gloves.*] Alright, I'll hold off on the Foley [catheter] and I can take a look at your skin. Would you say . . . can you describe the itch a little bit more to me? Is it just . . . you said it was annoying, is it painful or anything?
> JASON: No, it's just literally itchy.

---

3. A primary risk of deep vein thrombosis, the blood clot that students discover in Jason's calf, is that it will detach from the veins and travel to his lungs, where it will become lodged in the pulmonary artery that supplies blood to the lungs. This results in a life-threatening pulmonary embolism.

SEAN: [*Uses both hands to feel neck on both sides.*] Itchy around your neck? [JASON: Mhm.] And your stomach you said? [JASON: Mhm.] Do you mind if I take a look?

JASON: Almost kind of everywhere. Sure.

SEAN: [*Folds down the blanket so that Jason's torso is uncovered.*] I'm going to expose your stomach here. [*Lifts up the patient's dressing gown. Touches the top part of Jason's chest lightly with his right hand while he holds the dressing gown up with his left.*]. There is a little bit of, would you say it's bruising?

STEPHANIE: [*Walks from the medicine cart to the side of the bed next to Sean.*] That's from the accident.

JASON: Yeah, it's a little tender there. I have that seatbelt bruise.

STEPHANIE: [*Comes behind Sean to check the IV bags hanging from Jason's pump.*]

SEAN: [*Gently touches different spots around the torso.*] As I'm touching it, what are you—can you describe to me what you feel?

JASON: Well, it just feels like a bruise, you know.

SEAN: Sorry, your abdomen.

JASON: Oh. Oh, it's okay.

SEAN: It's okay? [JASON: Yeah] Does the itching get relieved when I touch it?

JASON: Uh no, not really. It doesn't make a difference.

SEAN: [*Turns to Stephanie, who is walking toward the medicine cart and reaches over to grab medication.*] What do we have for the . . . ?

STEPHANIE: [*Walking back toward the bed.*] So, I was reading that itching can be a side effect of the Lovenox [SEAN: Lovenox] Yeah. [*Walks back toward the medicine cart.*]

SEAN: [*Pulling Jason's gown back down and blanket back up over his torso.*] And is um, [*Gestures to the medication Stephanie is holding.*] that can heighten the . . .

STEPHANIE: [*Reading off the physician's orders at the medicine cart.*] Yeah, twenty-five milligrams IV push every six hours, yeah.

SEAN: So, Jason we've got, I don't know if you overheard our conversation. Stephanie was talking about how itching could be a side effect of the Lovenox that the previous shift gave you.

In this excerpt, students move around the physical space of the simulation room, apply sanitizer, put on exam gloves, check physician's orders at the medicine cart, and adjust the patient's blankets. All these movements provide opportunities to practice occupying a clinical space like a nurse and feeling the various physical sensations that accompany clinical care. Students also physically interact with the manikin, adjusting his dressing gown and touching his neck and chest, verbally narrating these actions when appropriate. In this way, the simulation setting offers affordances for practicing the physical body work of nursing. Simultaneously, the simulation environment enforces certain limitations on the nurse's body work. Sean mentioned in debrief his confusion with assessing the patient's skin when there were no visible symptoms. Because Maura decided to add the allergic reaction at the last minute, the only physical signs present on the manikin were those related to his accident (chest bruising).

Creating Tactile Fidelity

Physical differences between the manikin body and a human body can also create simisms during the simulation. For example, when inserting a catheter on Eliana, Ryan did not follow the proper technique of holding the patient's labia open with the nondominant hand while inserting the catheter tube with the dominant hand. In debrief, he explained that he had not thought to use one hand to hold the labia open because "it was already wide open." Thus, the manikin did not provide the visual cue needed to prompt proper physical intra-action. Reflecting on his experience with catheter insertion on Eliana, Ryan described how the imperfect simulator body disrupted his care: "It doesn't move like a person [. . .] like putting a catheter in a female, you would have them bend their own legs and spread their legs rather than you adjusting them and you have to be a lot more rough with the manikin."

In addition, while internal vital signs are controlled with the computer, so Maura can easily adjust things like heart rate, breathing, and pupil dilation, the manikin's surface is more difficult to change. With preparation ahead of time, Maura can add things like the bruises on his chest from the car accident and the blood clot. These simulated visual indicators of problems are often much more exaggerated than they would be in real life. For example, Eliana's infected wound is coated in greenish Vaseline and looks, frankly, terrible. The instructors and I had some laughs watching students' horrified reactions when they took off the bandage to reveal the greenish discharge.

Maura also spent several days perfecting the blood clot for Jason's leg. She joked to me, "Some people scrapbook on the weekends. I make wounds." She tried putting a tiny freezer pack into a cup of hot tea, but it exploded. Ultimately, she hand-sewed a small, microwaveable rice pack, which she would insert under his bandages in between the first and second groups in the simulation. Jason would ask to have the compression device[4] taken off his left leg because it was hurting. In response, groups of students, with varying levels of efficiency, would discover the warm clot and order an ultrasound to confirm that it was a deep vein thrombosis (DVT). For them to recognize the protrusion on the manikin's leg as a blood clot and carry out the appropriate course of action, the clot had to "feel" right, including being the right size, shape, and temperature. Thus, Maura's weekend crafting was not misplaced; perfecting the tactile experience of the clot helped to make it a realistic physical cue for students and scaffolded their patient sense when encountering future clots.

Visible in this example, then, is how the physical space of the simulation and the manikin body provide lessons in body work, but also how critical the instructor is in prompting the students' physical experiences. Since I was sitting in the instructor room behind a one-way mirror with Maura, I observed the way she would physically immerse herself in the patient's character. Just as she was teaching students to be responsive and intentional caregivers, her success as a facilitator depended on a deeply rhetorical and embodied immersion in the simulation scenarios themselves that helped her recognize the many routes for productive disruptions. Sometimes she would enact patient experiences, scratching her neck, for example, while the patient complained of itching. During a sensitivity test where a student was poking the simulator's foot with a pen, Maura had to stand up and strain to try to see when the poke was being delivered and respond. At the same time, because she always had her mouth to the patient microphone, Maura's involuntary physical responses became the patient's. When she sneezed, the students in the simulation would say "God bless you" to the simulator. When she yawned while a student was listening to heart sounds, he became concerned about the inconsistency of the patient's breathing. Thus, links and disconnects between Maura's body and the simulator's body were an important part of the simulation's rhetorical context and disruptions that prompted action. Maura's rhetorical responsivity—her immersion in both the verbal action of the simulation and the physical exchange—was a critical part of lessons in body work.

Overall, simulations teach students to move like nurses using the manikin for physical interaction, the tools in the simulation room, and the simulation

---

4. Sequential compression devices (SCDs) are inflatable sleeves that are put over a patient's calves. They are used to prevent blood clots, especially in patients who have just had surgery. SCDs improve blood flow using an attached air pump that inflates and deflates the sleeves in a rhythmic sequence to mimic the action of walking.

space. The simulation environment and the instructor's ministrations provide lessons in body work by prompting students to react to unexpected physical encounters and to experience the consequences of their physical interactions in immediate ways. Maura puts a good deal of time and energy into ensuring that physical cues in the simulation are authentic and can provide an approximation of patient sense on the job. Of course, a complete representation of reality is impossible. However, by returning to the materialist emphasis on intra-action, we can also recognize that the fact that the simulation creates imperfect bodily cues can be an advantage. These imperfect physical encounters are disruptive, but disruptions are a vital contributor to lessons in body work since they destabilize habitual action and prompt reflection.

Emotional Body Work: Performing and Internalizing Feelings

Just as students learn to effectively move around the clinical space and interact with the patient, they also learn to perform appropriate emotions for the clinical workplace, choosing the correct moments to leverage deep or surface acting in response to patient needs. As with physical body work, Maura played a role in orchestrating these lessons in emotional body work as well, especially to help students shift out of a task-oriented focus that often distracted them from social connections with patients. This task-oriented approach to care was common across groups and is a frequent challenge for new nurses. Maura even warned students about the likelihood of getting "tunnel vision" during simulations and encouraged them to take a step back when they felt they were getting bogged down in details.

In general, the nursing simulations are structured around a set of tasks that students need to accomplish—listed in the physician's orders—and thus, many students described interventions as getting in the way of providing more empathetic care. Michelle explained how the list of interventions could dominate a group's conversation: "It's kind of hard at the very beginning [to focus on the patient] when everyone's trying to figure out what to do. [. . .] You kind of forget that the patient's there." Similarly, Kira noted how in moments of crisis during the simulation, it was easy for a group to lose sight of the patient's emotional needs while they dealt with medical needs: "It was really good [the nurse] got to know about his heritage and his parents but then they completely disconnected [during the pulmonary embolism] and meanwhile he's over there [. . .] like, 'What is going on? Come talk to me!'"

Caring for a Crying Manikin

Ultimately, many students struggled to connect with Jason during his simulation, in part because there were many technical tasks to accomplish for a post-op patient with a developing blood clot. At the same time, however, the setup for Jason's scenario identifies several key social-emotional needs; he has just been in a car accident for drunk driving and totaled his father's car, which he is very nervous about. Upon further investigation, students will learn the accident occurred in the wake of a breakup from his longtime girlfriend. He is missing substantial amounts of school and is worried about catching up and about his parent's reaction to the accident.

One strategy Maura would use to counter students' task-focused care was to make Jason cry if she felt that his emotional needs were being ignored. Actual liquid could flow from the simulator's eyes, which would often surprise students. As one student explained during debrief, "With anyone else crying you'd see eyes welling up, puffy, but it was like, 'Oh okay, he's crying!'" Even though Jason's tears were not perfectly human, they disrupted student actions and redirected care encouraging emotional body work. For example, in the following exchange, a nursing student is taking Jason's pulse when he suddenly begins to cry:

> KYLIE: What's going on? Talk to me.
> JASON: I think it's all just starting to hit me. What happened.
> KYLIE: [*Grabs a tissue and dabs the tears.*] Yeah? Are you in any pain right now?
> JASON: Yeah, I'm hurting a little bit, but mostly I'm just starting to worry about everything.
> KYLIE: What are you worried about?
> JASON: Well, you may have heard that when I had the [car] accident, I was drinking and I've never even been in trouble. I just haven't been in trouble before and never ever had a problem and I don't know how mad my dad's going to be.
> KYLIE: Do you want me to call your dad and we can talk to him? We can have him come in.
> JASON: [*Exhales.*] I'm just not ready to face [my parents] so no, thank you, but not yet.
> KYLIE: Of course, is there anyone else you want to talk to?
> JASON: I don't know, I just—I don't know if I can go back to school, I just don't know a whole lot of stuff. It's just all hitting me what happened and I just can't [inaudible].

KYLIE: I know. It's okay. We're just going to get you well and then you can focus on it once you feel better, okay? Is there something I can do for you right now, though?

JASON: [*Exhales.*] No, just uh—you're right, I just have to focus on getting better.

KYLIE: That's okay, do you want to talk about it?

JASON: Well, go ahead and do whatever you have to do and I'll—I'm okay, thanks for listening. I'll be alright.

At the beginning of this conversation, Kylie tries to intervene to "fix" the crying. Kylie begins by assuming the crying male patient is suffering from physical pain. Once she discovers that the pain is emotional, she makes several offers to contact Jason's parents or others for support. Ultimately, though, Kylie realizes that Jason is just looking to talk about his feelings, and so her last offer is simply to listen. The exchange between Kylie and Jason is notable because the solution is to set aside instincts for identification or intervention and listen to the patient's experience from their point of view, a move that closely resembles "standing under," another tactic for rhetorical listening (Ratcliffe).

Ratcliffe emphasizes that "standing under" necessitates a shift from listening *for* a speaker's intent or our own interests to listening *with*. In this instance and undoubtedly many clinical contexts, the provider's automatic response is to listen *for* the problem so that they can identify an intervention. In fact, in Strekalova et al.'s research on empathetic communication in nursing, the most advanced mode of empathy is described as "identify[ing] actions that could enhance the patient's well-being" (71). Dearing and Steadman similarly link redirection of both feeling and situations to successful communication of nursing empathy (174).

However, Maura's disruption necessitates that Kylie listen *with* and let the patient's experiential "discourses wash over, through, and around" (Ratcliffe 28). A materialist lens also calls attention to the rhetorical role the simulator plays in fostering this exchange. The crying was a catalyst for Kylie's responsive intra-action. The imperfect tears, while not a replica of on-the-job patient sense, still provided a physical cue that worked in tandem with the coordinator's words to disrupt Kylie's agenda and foster a different kind of listening. Learning to dwell in the uncertainty of such moments helped students navigate between their premeditated, often static plans for a patient and the person's emergent needs, ultimately gaining the rhetorical skills to listen deeply and build greater connections with patient experience.

Documenting Body Work: Encoding Sensorial Encounters

In their investigation of a primary care clinic, Opel and Hart-Davidson find that although it is devalued by practitioners, writing is of paramount importance: "the most valuable thing that primary care clinicians produce is [. . .] a record of the body that can assist in caring for that body over time" (368–69). However, given that patient information is often gathered at an interface between patient and practitioner bodies, translating embodied knowledge into discursive documentation is not always straightforward. Mulla describes forensic nurses producing evidentiary rape records as "encod[ing] rich sensorial encounters [. . .] involving pain, odors, and bodily discourses" (24). In a similar way, nursing students must learn to encode knowledge gained from embodied interactions into their patient's medical chart so that they can become part of a "record of the body." The personal connections they build with patients, the intuitive knowledge they acquire from physical presence in a room with the patient (Campbell and Angeli), these inexpressible markers of patient sense must be somehow encoded to facilitate patient care and transfer.

While the focus of this section may seem distinct from previous sections because attention is on documenting the patient's body (i.e., a skin condition), all of this information has been gathered through bodily interactions between nurse and patient described in previous sections (i.e., palpating the skin). Thus, the nurse's body work is at the heart of their patient knowledge, which is part of what makes it challenging to discursively translate that embodied knowledge for others. I argue that a rhetorical view of body work emphasizes its relationship to written discourse, which has received less attention in sociological research.

In clinical simulations, all patient documentation was done on a large whiteboard in the center of the room. Prior to the start of the simulation, the full group of ten students would decide on a template for charting, including what categories to include and how to differentiate between each team's care. I have written about how these whiteboards provide an opportunity for students to negotiate prior genre knowledge and make strategic choices about how to design the simulated patient health record to best suit the simulation environment (Campbell, "Simulation Genres"). For the purposes of this chapter, the most relevant aspect of patient-chart design is its capacity to either normalize the patient exchange—keeping students task-focused and oriented toward the physician's orders—or to disrupt prior genre knowledge and encourage students to find new ways to document a patient's social and emotional needs.

The "To-Do" List

One group began their simulation with a huddle at the medicine cart, using the physician's orders and the previous groups' charting to create a "to-do" list that would guide their care of Jason. As Liz explained, "My group really right off the bat just like bam bam bam. We know what we have to do, let's get these things done, let's prioritize, have interventions that need to be done, and figure out the rest from there." The advantage of this documentation was easily apparent in this group's interactions with the patient and with one another throughout their simulation. They moved rapidly through orders, administering oxygen, giving two medications in rapid succession, providing food, and ordering an ultrasound for the patient's swollen leg. Not only that, but they were able to easily coordinate care across the members so that everyone was kept busy. Thus, the student-designed "to-do" list effectively coordinated student body work throughout the sequence, helping students work through feelings of anxiety, take up activities in different areas of the room to avoid crowding the patient, and overall move and talk in concert with one another.

Even in the observation room, Maura, the instructor, and I could feel the difference with groups like this, where care felt seamlessly sequenced. Maura described another group who was similarly well coordinated as "dancing" during their debrief, saying, "You guys were quiet, but you danced. You moved into place and got things done." This metaphor speaks to the way that instructors and students alike could feel the rhythm of an effectively designed chart as it enabled students to move efficiently through the simulation space and to expertly sequence patient care, a coordination that felt seamless.

That said, the chart's limitation was that its task-focused orientation allowed for less flexibility in responding to the patient's needs as they emerged organically over the course of the simulation. The group took a long time to discover Jason's blood clot in his left leg and needed multiple promptings from Maura, both because they were busy moving through other tasks on their list and because they wanted to keep the compression devices on his legs on to keep this item checked off their list. For most groups, Jason's mention of pain in his left leg was enough of a prompt for a student to take off the compression device to investigate the leg more closely. In this group, however, Jason's mention of pain led to a longer exchange:

> JASON: Can I ask you something though? [CARL: Yeah.] Can we take that squeezy thing off my leg? It's kind of bugging me.
> CARL: The SCDs? [JASON: Yeah.] Well we just turned them on and they're for your—[*Walks around from the right-hand foot of the bed where he has*

been looking at the catheter bag to the left-hand head of the bed so he can talk to directly to the patient. Liz comes over on the right-hand side with her head turned toward the patient, listening in.] we're trying to prevent a blood clot from happening in your body. After a post-op one of the common problems is developing a blood clot in your lower extremities especially if you have trauma to your legs, which you have [JASON: Okay.] So it's really really preventative because if it causes a blood clot that can get really scary, it's really dangerous and so it's a really important preventative measure. [JASON: Oh.] And so we want to keep them on as often as we can. [JASON: Okay.] So I know that they are a little bit uncomfortable, but we could do periodic breaks with them.

JASON: Okay, can I just take one break on my, just my left, you can leave on the other one it's just . . .

CARL: The left one? [JASON: Yeah.] Okay. [*To Liz*] How long do you think we could do a break on one of those?

LIZ: Um, I don't know.

JASON: I mean I guess if it's a big deal I can deal with it.

CARL: Okay, well are you in pain with it? Is it causing you pain or is it just discomfort?

JASON: Yeah, it's kind of hurting but I'll just—I'll push my button and see if that helps.

CARL: Okay, okay. If it increases then we'll definitely take it off, okay? Just keep—just let us know. [*Walks away from the bed.*]

Notably, Carl did not just dismiss Jason's complaint but instead offered a thorough explanation of the rationale behind the compression devices and their necessity given Jason's recent operation. By the end of his explanation, he even offers Jason a "break" from the devices, checking in with another student about how long they could take them off for. However, he does not ask Jason about specifics of the pain (what level it is; what it feels like), nor does he use the complaint as a prompt to physically investigate the leg further. When Jason offers to keep enduring the pain, Carl is quick to move on to the next task on their list. It is not until Jason starts softly moaning several minutes later that the group takes off the compression device and discovers the blood clot.

This example demonstrates how the design and implementation of their patient chart in simulations was not static for students. Even a chart that was designed to be responsive to the simulated context and beautifully coordinated student body work was not always able to capture emergent knowledge and facilitate patient empathy effectively. And, in fact, this chart could act as an impediment to acquiring additional patient knowledge. It could keep students moving forward rather than encouraging them to take off the compression cuff, touch the leg, feel the warmth of the blood clot, and revise their care, and maybe even their charting, accordingly.

Capturing Emotional Knowledge

In contrast to the "to-do" list, other groups worked to modify the constraints of the whiteboard patient chart to better capture knowledge about the patient's emotional experience. For example, in one group, Jason called the nurses over to request that they let him talk to his mom before his dad about his car accident. The students worked to accommodate this information into their chart design, which had been organized around "systems" in the right-hand column (neurological, respiratory, etc.). One student drew a small box in the left-hand corner of the board labeled "Pt" [Patient] that included the categories "Q?" [Question], "Task:" and "Note:." Under "Note" she wrote: "Can we only have his mother come into the room" (see figure 2 on the next page). While many teams did not document this conversation on the board at all, this team modified their chart to note the information, although with little additional context. In this way, they navigated a greater limitation of the professional genre—its inability to capture emotional patient experiences and knowledge.

In his discussion of how genres mediate interpersonal relationships, Bawarshi argues that the patient medical form's focus on physical over mental experiences shapes the encounter between physician and patient, causing the doctor to "treat the patient as a synecdoche of his or her physical symptoms" (74). Similarly, nursing faculty in Ariail and Smith's study expressed concern that the formulaic nature of the health record might prevent students from documenting vital patient information, like listing a frail patient's weight and height but "neglecting to include any discussion of psychosocial issues that impact eating habits of the patient" (247). Therefore, scholars have found that the sections and categories that organize professional patient health records support symptom-focused exchanges between patient and healthcare provider rather than facilitating empathetic connection with patient experience.

Similarly, this example demonstrates that even student charts that were designed to be responsive to the simulation context could carry with them the vestiges of a professional genre's constraints. Even though their simulation health records were not designed to prioritize emotional patient information, the students in this example still acted flexibly within their design to document more than physical symptoms. Because students are using their

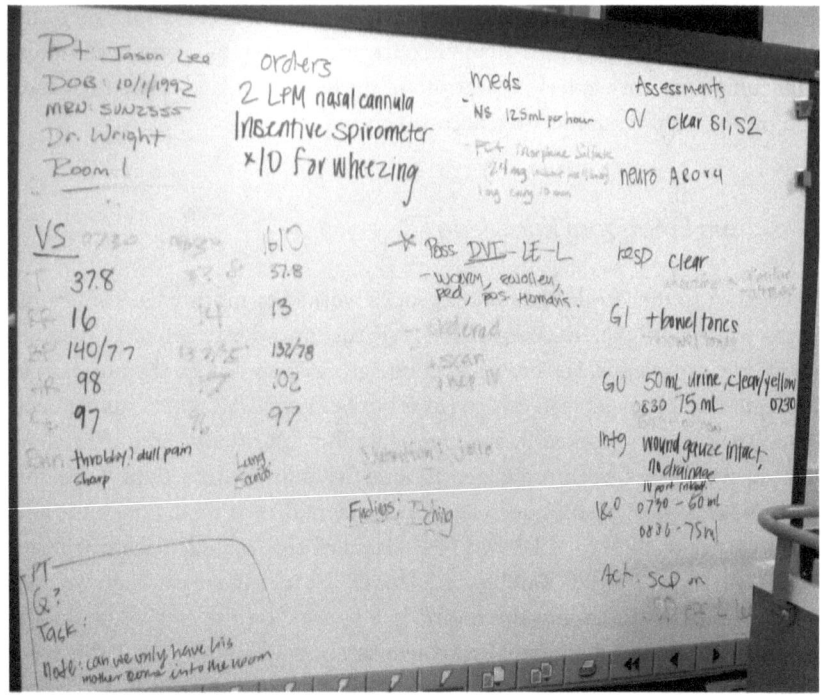

FIGURE 2. Interpersonal patient information charted by students on a simulation room whiteboard. Photo by author.

own records to guide care, the simulation context provides opportunities for them to experience firsthand how different choices can constrain the documentation of their embodied knowledge and to innovate in response to these limitations.

Finally, when miscommunications happened in simulations, the patient chart could also become a site where misinterpretations in body work were carried across groups. For example, during a pediatric simulation one group asked about infant Eric's skin. Maura responded that it was "warm and moist," intending to indicate that it was normal. However, the students misinterpreted this response to mean that the baby was sweating. This was another instance of a simism, where artificial aspects of the simulation context interrupted student care. These students later determined that Eric's blanket felt wet as well and during a phone call to the physician described the baby as "sweating profusely." On the board, under "Skin" they wrote "Warm/Moist," and also listed under "Plan," "Keep pt [patient] dry and comfortable." During the debrief, their instructor clarified that the baby was not, in fact, sweating but his blanket was just moist from coughing up formula. The debrief provided students and instructors an opportunity to both recognize those misinterpretations and become aware of how knowledge could become crystallized in the patient's record. In this way, the body work of an individual nurse moves from being an isolated sensory experience to shared patient knowledge.

A Troublesome Example

Having considered how lessons in rhetorical body work—physical, emotional, and discursive—manifest during a clinical simulation, I now want to turn to an example where all three of these elements came together during a problematic patient exchange. This example shows how several of the physical and emotional cues in the simulation designed to approximate the patient sense of a hospital room—including the patient manikin, the patient preparation sheet, and the simulation room—can intra-act to culminate in a problematic moment of cultural insensitivity.

It was the last round of a simulation caring for Jason Lee, and the third team of students was clearly on edge because simulations typically followed a trajectory where they increased in intensity with each group. Alice, who had a Chinese background herself, had really latched onto Jason's assumed Chinese heritage, garnered from the image on the preparation sheet and from his last name. In fact, she put the instructor Maura's cultural knowledge to the test in an early exchange when she asked Jason about his favorite Chinese New Year snack. Maura was fumbling around for an answer when a student assistant in the performance lab happened to walk by the simulation backroom and offer "moon cakes" as a suggestion.

As the pulmonary embolism caused Jason to begin struggling to breathe, he turned to Alice for reassurance. "What should I do?" he asked her. Alice again picked back up on their shared cultural heritage. "Think about . . . think . . . imagine that you're Buddha," she stammered. And continued on: "You're Buddha. Imagine that you're Buddha. Imagine—you know how he stayed underneath that tree for forty-nine days? [Yeah.] Just imagine that just, channel your inner, inner Buddha."

This exchange shows the challenges for a new nurse in navigating the difficult emotional terrain of patient panic as Jason's health rapidly deteriorates. In addition, it demonstrates how one nurse attempted to connect emotionally with a patient through shared cultural background. Focal students noted how this moment felt uncomfortable for observers because it seemed presumptuous to talk about religion without knowledge of Jason's beliefs. However, Alice was actively immersed in the simulation and working to calm Jason down. She was both modulating her own emotional reaction to the stressful situation and managing the patient's emotional state to the best of her ability. To push this emotional work further, Maura prompted Alice to provide physical comfort as well by having Jason respond to her discussion of Buddha with "Will you hold my hand?"

In the final moments of this simulation, Jason was being transferred to the intensive care unit and was still struggling to breathe. A bit of joking had already ensued with the respiratory therapist (the clinical instructor), and Alice left Jason with the comment "Imagine Buddha, but not too hard. Don't go to Buddha." Here, the facade of the simulation had been removed and the cultural reference that had served as a point of connection between patient and nurse became a source of humor about his death. The instructor laughed and touched Alice affectionately on the shoulder, making it clear that she and the student had removed themselves emotionally from the simulated context and were now transitioning back into "classroom mode."

In an interview, focal student Kira, who had been watching this simulation with the rest of the class from another room, mentioned Alice's interactions when I asked whether she remembered anything about other groups' communications with Jason. She responded, "Yes. Yes. Go to Buddha," indicating that this had been a memorable and problematic moment. Kira attributed the awkwardness to the simulation context: "I think they just got thrown off by the Sim and it just—it just went so bad." I did not press further, but Kira appeared to share in my experience of these comments as jarring and inappropriate. The joke's cultural insensitivity coupled with the dismissiveness about death made it an upsetting moment that seemed to undermine patient–nurse relations and the capacity for patient empathy.

Despite its troublesome nature, one could argue that the capacity to find humor in the face of death is a necessary emotional skill for a future nurse, one that distances her from her patients, yes, but also enables her to continue to perform emotional body work. Hochschild warns about the detrimental effects of constantly suppressing emotions in workplace contexts, noting that humor is often one way to navigate these emotions (*Managed Heart* 79). Similarly, reflecting on his experiences of joking during a town-wide anthrax simulation, Magelssen argues that humor is productive in its capacity to strengthen participant relationships: "The laughter likely fostered the kind of goodwill and camaraderie that drove home for participants how much they valued their hometowns, families, and social networks" (137). For Magelssen, flexibility and willingness to embrace disruptive moments that step outside of the simulation scenario can help support community building and camaraderie.

Thus, humor among students as they negotiate the boundaries between the real and the simulated might provide necessary emotional release and reinforce in-group identity for the burgeoning professionals. But humor becomes problematic when it overshadows the important learning about emotional modulation that is a focus of lessons in body work. Singer begins an article with a similarly troubling anecdote about a group of nursing students laughing after arranging a simulated body so that the top half is male and the bottom half is female. He argues, "The laughter of these students, if neither purposeful nor malicious, reveals that trans-specific embodiment is unthinkable, hence invisible, in clinical settings" (250). In both examples, shared levity is troublesome when it reinforces stereotypes about nonnormative body types or cultures and disregards empathetic exchange. These emotional lessons are further complicated by the distance between the facilitators in simulations and the demographics of the patients they represent, as evidenced by Maura's inability to respond to the Chinese New Year question. This distance points to the need for more direct engagement with diverse cultures in both the design and the enactment of clinical simulations, an argument that Press makes in her article about standardized patienthood as well.

A primary critique of clinical simulation is that by replacing human patients with robotic manikins, simulations have the potential to further support a standardization of bodies in medical practice and a lack of responsiveness to individual patient needs. However, this critique exists on the premise that simulators are merely acted upon, rather than seeing them as rhetorical actants in their own right. It is also built on the assumption that the learning in clinical simulations is skill-focused and assimilation-oriented. When we look at the simulator and nursing simulation environment in action we see that, in fact, there are many disruptive forces within this context that require regular attention, engagement, and responsiveness from students and that open up possibilities for critical discussion and revision of practice. In direct contrast to these critiques, the manikins and simulation environments demand a kind of radical responsiveness and radical situatedness to negotiate everything from a large manikin body that is nearly impossible to reposition to a face that unexpectedly starts leaking tears.

Certainly, the manikin bodies are not perfectly human, and the intra-actions that students have with them are regularly disrupted both intentionally by the instructor and unintentionally by quirks of the environment and manikin. However, these disruptions provide students opportunities for reflection as they identify and discuss how their practices will change and adapt in a clinical setting. Disruptions ensure that differences between contexts are at the center of students' lessons in body work during clinical simulations, which positions them as critical and engaged learners rather than merely receivers of static technical knowledge. In addition, there is a great deal of ambiguity in what students see, hear, and feel in simulations, and many of them can recognize how this lack of clarity will reflect their real-world encounters with ambiguity in clinical settings. In this way, their experiences of patient sense as muddled and uncertain reflects the experience of a novice in clinical settings. Meanwhile, willingness to consult others, reassess and revise their care, and stay attentive to new cues will serve them well on the job.

With all of that in mind, this chapter also suggests that there is more work to be done in leveraging nursing simulations to teach cultural responsiveness and attention to differences like race and class, alongside emotional performances like empathy. Body work and the notion of patient sense demonstrate how the troublesome moment I described emerges at an intersection of physical, emotional, and discursive learning that is generated by the particularities of the simulation context. This example also points to a range of ways that instructors might better prepare for such encounters, including (1) considering openly with students the discursive cuing around race, gender, and class that is occurring in the preparation sheets they receive and how that cuing will inform care; (2) deciding what kinds of experiential knowledge the instructor needs to effectively engage in conversations that touch on cultural, racial, or gendered backgrounds and using available resources to garner that knowledge; and (3) asking students to constellate possibilities for care during debrief conversations by considering together how their care might shift for a patient with a different background (Campbell, "Simulating Gender").

This analysis also points to the vital role of instructors in shaping students' body-work acquisition, lest anyone express a view that the use of robots in healthcare training should lead to the removal of human instructors. Maura was a fundamental part of the simulation's success, not just in facilitating action but also in cuing students' connection-making to the professional world and calling their attention to the multiplicity of possibilities for action. As I demonstrated, she was often as physically and emotionally immersed in the simulation as her students, and that level of engagement brought both authenticity and stakes to students' performances. The success of Maura's facilitation points to the many ways that instructors can create an environment in which students are able to position themselves in new rhetorical contexts and practice the physical, emotional, and discursive learning that will accompany their future roles. And her vital role previews the important influence of the physical therapy instructor in the next chapter, who critically shaped students' body work through stories of work in the field.

CHAPTER 3

More Than a Massage

Body Work as Boundary-Work in a Physical Therapy Lab

A casual observer happening upon the physical technologies lab at Midwest University on any given afternoon might find themselves more than a little shocked and concerned. One day, they could encounter students sprawled out on patient beds around the room, sticking electrode pads to one another's upper arms, calves, and backs and delivering electrical stimulation via a small penlike remote. Another day, they might discover students lying prone on their backs while another student taps a needle into their arm and wiggles it around, practicing a dry needling technique used to provide relief to tense muscles. They could find students rubbing ultrasounds over one another's extremities or competing to see who could get their partner's arm to involuntarily raise the highest with an electrical shock.

In these moments, physical therapy students are acquiring lessons in body work at the technology interface, learning how technologies can mediate patient sense in their future professions. They are also practicing emotional and verbal modes of body work, moderating their peers' anxiety and pain in response to technological interventions. As they activate knowledge from their textbooks and lectures in the lab, physical therapy students begin to take on professional identities. This is a process which is particularly fraught in a field that regularly must assert its domain of professional expertise. Meanwhile, the stories that circulate in the lab and the ad hoc conversations during care make up the hidden curriculum of students' education—unwritten rules and logics of a discipline that are as central to its professional identity as textbooks and competency checklists (Witman). As I discovered during my observations in the physical technologies lab, rhetorical body work in physical therapy is embodied boundary-work, geared toward reinforcing the field's scientific knowledge base and expertise while distancing it from feminized or sexualized contexts.

Most people who have received care from a provider in the "touch professions," like physical therapy, occupational therapy, or chiropractic care, would agree that the body-to-body contact in these contexts is skilled, representing a good deal of training and expertise. And yet, practitioners in these fields have had to fight to assert their professional status and domain, distinguishing themselves from individuals who might claim a title without the training (George). Their struggles show the way that grounding professional practice in physical exchange between practitioner and patient is also precarious. Centering embodied practice has the potential to undermine perceptions of scientific expertise and to threaten a profession's standing, affiliating it instead with feminized care domains or sex work (Wolkowitz, *Bodies*). This is likely why Wainwright et al., in their research on mothers learning massage and reflexology, find "the body and its corporeality come second to [an] emphasis on science" (84). Burgeoning professional fields must work harder to clearly establish and delineate their scientific expertise while distancing themselves from the kinds of professional denigration that can come from affiliation with feminized or sexualized contexts.

Thus, the history of physical therapy is one of navigating its professional role in relation to other practitioners—nurses, doctors, occupational therapists, chiropractors—some that have attained professional recognition and status and others that have been relegated to the realm of complementary and alternative medicine (CAM). Scholars have found that professions like physical therapy must choose their allegiances carefully. Alliances with Western biomedical frameworks require standardization of practices that often fundamentally rely on individualized interventions (Derkatch 47) but also bring legitimization through accreditation and insurance coverage of treatment (Moffat 22).

Overall, physical therapy is an allied health field that, at least within the United States, has largely succeeded in establishing itself as a distinct, biomedical health profession. This has been demonstrated through the spread of doctoral programs and field-specific journals, as well as PTs' autonomy in patient diagnosis and treatment (Moffat). Still, PT professionals face the constant risk of professional denigration through persistent bodily contact. It is certainly more challenging to cordon off the body into parts (Wolkowitz, "Social Relations" 501) for someone responsible for muscular rehabilitation than for a cardiologist or a gynecologist. As a result, physical therapy courses do the disciplinary work of assimilating students into a unique professional ethos while they are also learning to navigate embodied strategies and technological tools within the profession.

This chapter draws on six weeks of observation in a physical therapy lab at a midsize private university in the Midwest to better understand the unique rhetorical body work that students are learning and its relationship to professional identity and ethos. After considering the importance of boundary-work for the allied professions, I briefly introduce the physical technologies lab and its practices. Next, I discuss the stories that circulate in the lab, both students' stories about their entrance into the field and practitioners' stories about previous patients. These stories work to establish professional ethos and inform body work, but at times they can also reinforce patient stereotypes and devalue patients' embodied knowledge, elements that work against the centrality of patient sense in physical therapy. From there, I unpack the physical learning in the lab, both body-on-body interactions and technologically mediated care. In both cases, students are gaining a burgeoning sense of patient experience through their partners' feedback. While physical encounters will make up the bulk of their future patient care, the emphasis on technologies in the lab environment both reinforces anatomical knowledge and cues students to their partner's reactions, preparing them to be responsive providers in the future. This offers crucial learning about physical body work but is also limited by both social dynamics and physical variation in the lab. Thus, in the conclusion, I consider the "hidden curriculum" in physical therapy and the potential risks of reinforcing patient stereotypes and gendered assumptions about professionalism.

Embodied Boundary-Work and the Allied Health Professions

Science studies has had an ongoing interest in how boundaries are drawn and maintained between scientific fields and nonscience, a process which occurs within the scholarly discourse of a discipline (Bazerman; Derkatch) but also in the everyday interactions between practitioners in a lab (Latour and Woolgar) or interprofessional collaborations (Wilson and Herndl). In his seminal work, sociologist Gieryn describes these efforts to demarcate science as boundary-work, defined as "attribution of selected characteristics to the institution of science (i.e., to its practitioners, methods, stock of knowledge, values and work organization) for purposes of constructing a social boundary that distinguishes some intellectual activities as 'non-science'" (781). Despite his positioning in sociology, Gieryn identifies boundary-work as a matter of rhetorical style, concerned with discursive framing of scientific and nonscientific pursuits. He also recognizes that identification as a "science" is not just a theoretical classification. It has direct material consequences: "Because of considerable material opportunities and professional advantages available only to 'scientists,' it is no mere academic matter to decide who is doing science and who is not" (781). This is even more true in the biomedical sciences, where demarcation as a science brings not just access to grants but also to insurance reimbursement for patients, making treatment accessible and expanding the reach of a profession significantly.

Building on this idea of boundary-work, several scholars have traced the struggles of allied health professions in the process of establishing their identity and legitimacy within biomedical frameworks. Derkatch analyzed a series of articles on CAM practices in the *Journal of the American Medical Association (JAMA)* archives, finding that the biomedical assimilation of CAM into *JAMA*'s frameworks brings about ideological contradictions for what counts as evidence and how procedures should be evaluated. Thus, "while many CAM interventions are individualized for specific patients [. . . they] are standardized when molded into a medical-scientific framework, consequently requiring that intervention to perform equally across populations" (47). Spoel and James describe a similar contradiction between quantitative and qualitative frameworks in their research on inclusion of midwifery as one of Ontario's self-regulated and self-funded health professions. They highlight the challenges of bringing a holistic profession that is grounded in second-wave feminist values of female autonomy and pregnancy as a state of health in line with biomedical frameworks. In response, midwives worked to distinguish themselves from other feminized professions like nursing while also emphasizing how their holistic approach to care was tied to their largely female pool of practitioners.

Visible in both the example of CAM and midwifery is the important role that patient sense plays in the allied health professions. Embodied, intuitive knowledge and direct encounters with individual patient bodies are central to how practitioners *know* in these fields, and assimilating that knowledge into biomedical frameworks is particularly challenging. Also visible in these examples is the valuing of the patient's own embodied knowledge. For example, CAM interventions are tailored to specific patients, and midwives prioritize female autonomy, demonstrating how both fields center patients' experiences and feedback. This is an approach that is often called for in work in rhetoric of health and medicine (RHM) and narrative medicine. RHM research on conditions like irritable bowel syndrome (Kessler), diabetes (Anderson; Jeffrey Bennett), and COVID-19 (Swacha) argues for the importance of centering patient stories, elevating the experiential knowledge that they bring of day-to-day experiences with disease or chronic conditions. While these perspectives are moving into more mainstream healthcare contexts through frameworks like patient-centered care, they have long been the norm for holistic health professions.

Alongside the need to quantify subjective, individualized care, burgeoning health professions also face the challenge of claiming a recognizable domain of knowledge and articulating a distinct professional identity. A 2013 physical therapy vision statement calls for the field to lay claim over "movement systems" as their domain (Sahrmann). Advocates argue that associating the field with a system gives them more professional status than identifying with a specific intervention, particularly because it creates opportunities to contribute to scientific knowledge-making. The call to focus on a movement system might in fact help explain how physical therapy's status has been achieved. Wolkowitz argues that "higher status occupations tend to see themselves dealing with a bounded body, partly through mapping it as a system, leaving lower status ones to deal with what is rejected, left over, spills out and pollutes" ("Social Relations" 501).

While research on boundary-work has primarily focused on discursive rhetoric, rhetorical body work calls us to investigate how boundary-work is also tied to embodiment. Wainwright et al.'s research on mothers' training in massage and reflexology, for example, shows how specific embodied practices are required to "professionalize" the massage students. The students are required to wear uniforms, which the authors argue "can be interpreted as providing a distancing mechanism from the bodily" (83). The women, who often enroll with the impression that massage and reflexology will draw on their "natural" feminine capacities as women and mothers, are also explicitly encouraged to tone down expressions of femininity. They are required to keep their nails short, wear their hair back, wear minimal makeup, and not wear any jewelry—requirements which often hold true for nurses as well (84). And while these requirements are associated with values of professionalism and cleanliness, students were aware of their desexualizing function as well, given the affiliations that often occur between massage and sex work: "One student indicated: 'you can wear a little bit of makeup but obviously don't overdo it' as not to encourage the arousal of heterosexual male clients" (84).

As the embodied examples from Wainwright et al.'s research demonstrate, directives for bodily comportment in training contexts might be explicit (i.e., "keep your nails short"), but the implications of those directives ("so that men won't associate your body work with sex work") are part of a hidden curriculum tied to disciplinary identity and legitimacy. Hidden curriculum is a concept that has been explored in both sociology and education research, with consideration of its applications to medical education (Hafferty and Franks; Witman). Bourdieu's concept of the habitus is often associated with the hidden curriculum, as it constitutes a process of socialization leading to a shared professional identity that is internalized among students, "a system of dispositions: durable, subconscious schemes of perception and appreciation that activate and point the way to practice" (Witman 114). Importantly, hidden curriculum can foster professional identities that simultaneously stereotype or scapegoat other individuals. For example, Trainor demonstrates how a rural public school's narratives about hard work and success create a dominant habitus that otherizes and blames minoritized individuals for their struggles.

This chapter builds on these findings about how scientific boundary-work happens both linguistically and through embodied strategies of dress and comportment. It also builds on previous research in medical education about how professional ethos is transferred through both structured curricular interventions and ad hoc interaction and exchange in clinical contexts. Overall, rhetorical body work was critical for physical therapy students as a form of embodied boundary-work that professionalizes the patient sense that is at the heart of their practice. Importantly, it was acquired both in explicit lessons and in the hidden curriculum of the lab.

A Brief History of Physical Therapy

To understand the embodied rhetorical lessons in boundary-work that I encountered in the physical therapy labs, it is also important to have disciplinary history of the field and its professional ethos. This section focuses on three themes in PT's evolution: its ambivalent relationship to feminization, development alongside polio epidemics and world wars in the United States, and relationship to evolving technological tools.

Ottosson points out that physical therapy has often been coded as feminine, not just because women primarily practiced it but also because it was viewed as a "semi-profession," which "lacks what gender scholars have identified as professional attributes with masculine connotations, such as a high degree of autonomy and a unique scientific body of knowledge" (434). However, he also argues that the feminine history of the field overlooks its historic origins in the Royal Central Institute of Gymnastics, founded in Stockholm, Sweden, in 1813 by Pehr Henrik Ling. Ottosson describes Ling's educational program as highly masculinized, "very military in its appearance, sometimes earning the label 'Swedish drill'" (457). He believes this masculine identity within the field has been suppressed, with histories beginning later and tracing PT's origins to the Chartered Society of Physiotherapy (CSP) in Britain.

While I acknowledge Ottosson's call for a more expansive history of the field, the British all-female CSP's formation in 1894 is still an important professional moment. This organization emerged specifically in response to public rumors that several respectable massage clinics were operating as brothels. The need to distinguish themselves from sex workers early on demonstrated the professional risks for members of a field so closely engaged with body work, particularly for female practitioners. While professional formation responded to different exigencies in the United States, the first professional PT organization begun in 1921 was also exclusively female and named the American Women's Physical Therapeutic Association. The group did decide to change their name in 1922, however, to the American Physiotherapy Association (APA), to recognize the role of male reconstruction aides in war rehabilitation programs (Moffat 17). Participants in these associations were graduates of either physiotherapy or physical education programs and had knowledge of both massage techniques and technological interventions, either electrotherapy or hydrotherapy.

Within the United States, two primary exigencies drove the growth of physical therapy as a field at the beginning of the twentieth century. The first was rising and falling poliomyelitis (polio) epidemics, which began in Boston, Massachusetts, in 1893 and would continue until the vaccine became widespread in the 1950s (Moffat). In his article on polio's impact on professional formation in PT, Neumann discusses several important features of the disease. The most influential was polio's "spotty and random pattern of muscle paralysis," which meant that it was not uncommon for patients to lose function of only one or two muscles within a muscle group (488). This inconsistent paralysis caused polio clinics to become "virtual spawning ground[s] for lessons in kinesiology" (488), creating the foundation for PT to claim the movement system as its domain of expertise many decades later (Sahrmann). PTs could also make very notable progress with patients because many had continued muscle sensation surrounding their paralysis and thus could learn to activate adjacent muscles to regain normal function. Both patients and physical therapists could witness a very clear cause-and-effect relationship between their efforts and their accomplishments, which Neumann attributes to an overall optimistic and positive attitude within the field (485).

World Wars I and II also created a need to care for injured soldiers both at home and abroad, leading to the growth of PT. Following shortly after the US's entrance into World War I in 1917, Marguerite Sanderson was hired as director of the Reconstruction Aide program, and she began a training program at Walter Reed General Hospital to prepare reconstruction aide workers for overseas duty (Moffat 16). Growth was rapid—by 1919 forty-five hospitals around the country had physiotherapy facilities employing over seven hundred reconstruction aides. And while most of these aides were women, Linker also argues that the field had an ambivalent relationship to its feminine identity in this early period. In her view, "Physiotherapy represents a different kind of female professionalism—one that concerned itself more with achieving autonomy from other white-collar women than it did with gaining independence from white-collar men" (106). This may, in part, have been due to the attitudes toward and expectations for women working in the sciences during the wars.[1]

In her examination of early physical therapists, Linker finds that their masculine professional personas were not just discursive but also embodied, designed to highlight "their unique combination of brains and brawn [that] gave them authority over the disabled body" (106). This perspective represented a direct departure from other feminized professions like nursing, which specifically relied on female traits like compassion, nurturing, and physical gentleness. Instead, early PT professionals eschewed Victorian notions of womanhood, working to distance themselves from other white-collar women through alignment with male physicians. As Linker explains, "physiotherapists did not seek support from women's clubs or female associations for professional uplift; rather, physiotherapists legitimized their profession almost solely by association with the medical profession" (106). Overall, these endeavors were successful, with the field gaining increasing legitimacy and independence in the United States from the 1940s through the 1980s.[2]

That is not to say, however, that this period was without challenges. The field did experience an increase in the number of men entering the profession after World War II. This provided more continuity in staffing and increased wages and independence, which women PTs benefited from as well (Stiller 12). Still, the fight for legitimacy continued. Sahrmann describes her experience in the 1960s performing patient care under observation from a representative of the US Department of Labor who was working to determine whether physical

---

1. While women's professional participation in the sciences increased substantially in the early 1900s, women still struggled with the cultural valuing of rationality that dominated scientific spaces. In *Science on the Home Front,* Jack describes several female scientists during World War II and their efforts to participate in scientific norms of communication.

2. See Moffat's "The History of Physical Therapy Practice in the United States" for details. Highlights included the passage of the Hill Burton Act in 1946, which expanded hospital-based practice, the 1954 development of a seven-hour professional competency exam for state licensing boards, and a 1975 law which required schools to accommodate children with disabilities and moved PTs into education. In the 1980s, the United States dissolved the requirement that patients have a physician referral for PT, thereby recognizing the field's professional autonomy.

therapists were technicians or professionals (1035). Part of the struggle for professional ethos, then, was PT practitioners' regular interactions with technological tools that could position them in a technician role. As mentioned, one early criterion for members of the AWPTA was that they have experience with either electro- or hydrotherapy techniques in addition to massage. By the 1980s, practitioners were receiving pushback for what Moffat describes as "modality-pushing," which was being exorbitantly billed as PT began to receive insurance coverage under programs like Medicaid. With administration of a hot pack costing the same as physical techniques like massage, PTs saw the need to emphasize their expertise and "slowly began downgrading the fee for unattended modalities and drastically upgrading the fees for therapeutic exercise, functional training, and manual therapy" (Moffat 22).

Overall, several key themes emerge from this history that will be relevant to my consideration of the intersections between professional learning in PT and rhetorical body work. The first is the field's ambivalent relationship to a feminine identity. Ottosson's and Linker's thoughtful analyses of gendering in the field demonstrate its complex disciplinary terrain. On the one hand, the field does still hold on to a shared feminine history based in rehabilitation efforts during the world wars, but that is complicated both by alternative histories of PT's origins and through female professionals' efforts to distinguish themselves from other feminized allied health professions of the time. Second, the field's relationship to polio epidemics is crucial in understanding both its domain of expertise (the movement system) and its positive orientation. And third, the field's relationship to technology remains complex. From the beginning, it has touted technological expertise as a key component of professional PT knowledge. And yet, it has also frequently seen the risk of that relationship to technology relegating PT professionals to the role of technician. Since my fieldwork took place specifically in a physical technologies lab, this ongoing tension was visible and important to my findings about how students and instructors navigated rhetorical body work and performances of professional expertise.

Field Context

The Physical Therapy Lab

This research began with a conversation with the chair of the Physical Therapy Department at Midwest University. After discussing my interest in embodied communication in the health sciences, she recommended a class called

Physical Technologies as a research site. In her view, the physical technologies lab is the first place where PT students are guaranteed to be practicing the physical interactions that will be the basis for their future practice. This includes massage techniques as well as different modalities like hot and cold packs, ultrasound, dry needling, and electrical stimulation. After securing internal funding for the project, I reached out to the clinical instructor of Physical Technologies and offered him a stipend to participate in my research during his six-week summer course.

While there was some variation in the organization of the physical therapy lab depending on the activity, they generally began with fifteen to twenty minutes of instructor-led lecturing and demonstration followed by time for students to practice interventions on their partner. Sometimes students were asked to rotate through several partners, while other days they worked primarily with the same partner and switched off who was giving and receiving treatments. Lectures typically referenced anatomical learning that was taught earlier that day during the formal lecture but focused primarily on the interventions students would be practicing as well as contraindications (conditions that might prevent treatment). Occasionally, the instructor would call the students back together toward the end of the lab to practice documentation.

To be honest, while I was convinced early on that the physical technologies lab was the right location for me to be studying, I was not sure going into my study *how* I would collect data in the space. I did plan to video record, since my experiences with the simulation study had proven that video recording was vital for studying embodied learning. However, the lab consisted of a large, open floorplan, scattered with rolling, backless chairs, and massage tables with face holes for students to sit or lay down on while receiving care. Since thirty to thirty-five students participated in each lab, spread out all over the room, it was impossible for me to capture everyone giving and receiving care during the approximately ninety minutes of practice time. Initially, I thought that I might just follow a couple of students through their lab experiences. However, I was lucky to receive funding to provide stipends to student participants, which meant that I ended up having twenty-nine students interested in conducting a pre- and post-interview with me about their experiences in the lab.[3]

Given the large number of participants and the sprawling and chaotic layout of the lab, I ultimately decided that my goal was to video record each of my participants both providing and receiving care during the six-week

---

3. I asked several demographic questions at the beginning of my pre-interviews. Based on their responses, I had eight men and twenty-one women in the study; one participant identified as Black and three identified as Asian, while the remainder (twenty-five) identified as white.

course. Since partners would frequently switch during a single session, this typically meant I could stick with one pair of participants and get both the giving and receiving practice recorded. During pre-interviews, I learned more about students' personal and professional backgrounds and their views of the field. During their post-interviews, in addition to asking about their general experience in the course, I selected a two-minute clip of them either giving or receiving care and had them watch it. Then, I asked several specific questions about what they observed, including:

- Can you describe for me what's happening in this clip?
- What skills/techniques are you demonstrating in this clip?
- What communication strategies are you demonstrating in this clip? (see appendix 2)

This approach draws on the multimodal discourse analysis method that Jaclyn Fiscus-Cannaday and I developed to study teachers' disciplinary embodiment (Campbell and Fiscus-Cannaday), which is informed by Norris's ethnographic research on German women's identity construction. In line with my interest in discursive body work and my method while studying simulations, I also concluded the second interview by looking at documentation that students had written for the course and discussing their writing experience together.

Overview of the Physical Technologies Course

Midwest University's Doctorate in Physical Therapy program is a highly ranked national program that accepts both high school applicants at the beginning of their undergraduate careers and students transferring into the doctoral program after receiving a baccalaureate degree elsewhere. Internal applicants complete their undergraduate degree in three years and begin doctoral PT coursework in their fourth year. They can be enrolled in a range of undergraduate majors including health science fields like biomedical sciences, biomedical engineering, exercise physiology, and physiological sciences and social science / language fields (psychology, sociology, Spanish language). The program graduates between fifty-five and seventy new PTs per year. The Physical Technologies course is a four-credit course that students take during the summer following their first full year of physical therapy curriculum. For internal students this is their fourth year at Midwest University; for transfer students it is their first year.

The instructor of the physical technologies lab, Kevin, was a clinical professor who had received his master's in physical therapy and his PhD in biomedical engineering at Midwest University. He was an adjunct faculty member for several years before becoming a full-time clinical professor almost two decades ago; he had also recently received a prestigious university-wide reward for teaching excellence. He taught both the lecture component of the course, which ran three mornings a week for two hours, and the lab portion, which ran three afternoons a week for two hours. He typically taught back-to-back lab sessions with half the students in the first section and half in the second section. For labs, he had an experienced PT, Megan, working as an assistant to circulate and observe students during their practice. He also occasionally brought in guest visitors to teach more niche techniques, like dry needling. I observed one lab session a day, since the activities repeated, but made sure to alternate which groups I observed to observe all students. I was present and video recording at all three days of lab sessions for the six weeks of the course's duration, totaling approximately thirty hours of observation and video data.

Overall, energy and enthusiasm levels in the physical technologies lab were high. Kevin typically had music on during the practice time, usually letting students select a station so that the latest hits would be thumping in the background of student conversation. Out of necessity, students showed up in athletic gear so that they could move easily and their partners could access their bodies; it was also summertime, so shorts and sandals abounded and many students came in on Monday morning with new tan lines. This lent a casual atmosphere to the labs that was markedly different from the effect of having students wear scrubs to their nursing simulations. I felt a bit out of place in the professional outfits I chose to wear, especially as Kevin dressed casually in khaki shorts and would joke frequently with students about his leather sandals, his "Birks." In general, Kevin was a casual and clearly well-liked instructor. He had many inside jokes with students and had children their age who were enrolled at Midwest University, so he was privy to university events and activities.

Aside from the casual atmosphere, however, physical technologies was also the first place where students were really practicing hands-on physical therapy, and their enthusiasm to finally be learning "real" PT techniques was palpable. Their first year of curriculum focused heavily on "building the base of our knowledge" as one student put it, including courses in gross anatomy, pharmacology, kinesiology, and pathophysiology. When I asked students what they expected to learn in physical technologies then, the relief to be focused on PT interventions was clear. "This is like what we're actually doing with patients, so it feels more clinic based," noted one student.

My Body on the Scene: Afternoon Neck Traction

It is the end of a Tuesday afternoon session midway through the physical technologies lab when Kevin asks me if I am willing to partner with a student, since they have odd numbers today. The students are practicing neck traction and effleurage, techniques that can be used to treat headaches in the general population and to help stroke victims recover sensation. I am paired with Dan, who is not one of the focal students in the study, so we have not had much interaction up to this point. I keep the camera running while I lay down on the bed face up and scoot my head to the edge. On a replay, I discover that his body is blocking mine for much of the treatment and our conversations are difficult to discern from those of the instructor and other students.

Dan's interactions with me are immediately more formal than the other student pairs. He starts off by mimicking client talk, "Okay, Lilly, so today we're going to do some neck traction." Meanwhile, Kevin instructs the students to take off their shirts for more immediate access to the neck muscles and the clavicle, but I am dressed in a button-up shirt and not wearing a sports bra, so I leave my shirt on. Dan checks in frequently to ask how things are feeling as he torques my neck back and forth with both hands and massages the scalene muscles along the side of my neck with his thumb, following Kevin's verbal direction. The care proceeds as he moves from working his thumb down the muscles in my neck to my collar bone. When Kevin directs partners to switch, Dan begins the series again, starting with the torquing of my neck, though by this point I feel we are both starting to relax.

Toward the end of the massage, Dan moves to massaging a knot at the back of my neck. A tingling sensation extends down my spine and out toward my fingers and toes. It spreads a pleasing warmth through my extremities. Since a big part of my role is to give Dan feedback, I assume that it would be helpful for him to know what I am feeling, and I try to explain. "Whatever you just did there made me feel all tingly," I tell him and then immediately realize that sounds kind of creepy. Meanwhile, he becomes concerned that I am in pain. "No, no, it felt good," I assure him. "Just like a tingling sensation down my spine, probably blood flow?" I thought he might have a technical understanding of what was happening, but he does not, so instead this feedback just moves us into an awkward silence (or at least what feels like one from my end) for the last several minutes of the massage. He wraps up and I assure him that I feel "very relaxed" before we both go our separate ways. I am reminded how intimate and vulnerable the rhetorical body work I have been observing and recording between students truly is, an aspect that is sometimes easy to forget when I am on the other side of a camera.

Narrative Identity Construction in Physical Therapy

One of the things that struck me early on in my interviews with students and observations of the physical therapy labs was the predominance of patient stories. During interviews, students frequently told me stories about their own experiences in PT, remembering their PT providers fondly and describing in detail the atmosphere of the clinic. At the same time, while nursing simulations were structured around a single extended patient narrative, the physical therapy labs instead integrated patient stories alongside practice. Instructors would tell stories both during the instructional portion of the lab, while they demonstrated techniques, and as they walked around and supervised students practicing the technique. A key component of Kevin's co-instructors' role was to bring in perspective from the "real world" to help give student practice meaning and efficacy. Stories also dominated the in-between moments of lab work, so that several times I found a story in my field notes that I could not locate in my video recording because Kevin or another instructor shared it during a break or a transition.

Most stories in the lab concluded with a moral, a takeaway summary statement that the instructors would use to tie the narrative back to student action and intervention. In these morals, we also see the seeds of professional identity construction and field-specific boundary-work. As Detweiler and Peyton explain in their discussion of narrative within a new occupational therapy doctorate program, "When they gain the strength of numbers, the little narratives of experience exert a steady pressure on the metanarrative traditions of the field." In this section, I consider both the little narratives that students told about their discovery of PT and those that appeared in the in-between moments of lab to be components of what scholars have called the hidden curriculum in the classroom. I discuss the relationship between these little narratives and the larger messages being conveyed about physical therapists' identity and the professional field. I also demonstrate that while these narratives are primarily discursive, they have clear implications for the body work of PT professionals—offering them explicit guidelines on bodily comportment and engagement. This relationship between professional narratives and embodied practice is an area that has been underexplored and is a key component of understanding rhetorical body work.

Origin Stories: Choosing Physical Therapy

My first question for students in their pre-interview was why they had chosen to become a physical therapist. It quickly became apparent from their responses that there was a kind of origin story within the field that was typical. Many students had been former high school athletes who suffered a serious injury and found themselves on the receiving end of physical therapy. Marcia's story is typical: "In high school, I tore my ACL, so I was the actual patient for that and that was really interesting. I had a really good PT who would explain to me why he was doing what he was doing and why things hurt." This origin story was so well known that students were aware of the trope and would comment on it, either aligning their interest with the trend or recognizing themselves as outliers.

While certainly those heading into other health professions might have shadowed or talked to those working in the field, this widespread level of experience as a patient under the care of a PT seems exceptional. It means that many PT students are already arriving with experiential and embodied knowledge of what it feels like to be a PT patient, knowledge that undoubtedly shapes their understanding of patients' experiences during their care and, ultimately, their patient sense. Most of the students in the cohort I observed had personally received physical therapy care and usually had a pretty good time in the process. Reminiscing on her time in PT as a patient, Kelsie noted, "Me and my first PT, we would have laughs and make jokes during the session and it was enjoyable. I didn't feel like I do when I go to the regular doctor. It's kind of more sterile and a lot more transactional and professional." This sense of enjoyment was shared by many interviewees as well, with several students noting that they had chosen physical therapy because they could not imagine themselves at a desk job or because they considered themselves to be a "people person." Mika noted of her experiences receiving PT and shadowing in an office, "They all seem to really enjoy their jobs. Yeah, it's something you don't see in every field." Mika's and Kelsie's reflections tie back to Neumann's claim about PT's optimistic orientation as a field. They also reflect some of the bodily expectations that students bring to their training as physical therapists—that they will exude a cheery, positive attitude in their interactions with patients and one another, an expectation that was reflected in the atmosphere of the physical technologies lab as well.

Beneath the surface of a number of these claims about the fun side of PT, however, was a recognition that it was not considered to be as rigorous or serious as other medical fields. Several students commented that they had begun as premed or pre-pharmacy but had transitioned into PT because of the difficulty of those programs. For example, Michael noted: "I kind of figured out through college chemistry that pharmacy might not be for me, so then I started venturing out and looking into other things." Similarly, Kyle commented that he was "never good at math" as part of his explanation for pursuing the field. Still, there were several students who attributed their talent for science or their interest in anatomy as key to their career choice, especially those who were more academically oriented, working in a pain lab on campus or involved in neuroscience research collaborations.

Overall, a number of the students in my study came to physical therapy as a second resort. Sometimes this had to do with fears about the rigor of medical school, because they "heard that the MCAT was big and bad and scary," as one student put it, or "didn't necessarily want to go to Med school for you know 12 years or whatever," as another student explained. Other times, it was because their initial aspirations to be an athlete had fallen through. I note this not because I think it's atypical; most people will change career goals over the course of their college studies.[4] However, these prior experiences undoubtedly shape how practitioners in physical therapy orient more broadly to other medical professionals. Since many of them came into the field with perceptions that this was the easier or more fun route, there is a bit of a chip on their shoulder about the seriousness of the work. This came through not only in student conversations during my observations but also in the ways that instructors talked about other medical professionals and asserted their expertise.

At the same time, students articulated several clear advantages that PTs held over other medical professions, including time spent with patients and the ability to provide more holistic care. When I asked students what they believed to be unique about the PT's perspective as part of a medical team, almost all of them mentioned the extended patient relationships that PTs can build. For example, Sara commented, "With a nurse or a doctor, especially with your pediatrician or something like that, you see him once a year. With

---

4. See Angeli and Campbell, "Designing," for a discussion of incorporating winding career paths into writing in the health professions pedagogy.

PT you could see someone almost every day of the week depending on what they are [working on]. So you really get to build good rapport." Indeed, it was precisely these close relationships with their PT providers in high school that motivated many students to pursue the profession.

Along similar lines, students noted that these ongoing relationships meant that treatment was not just a one-off intervention but was about helping people develop new habits of movement that would improve their health long-term. As Lisa explained, "Sometimes you go in [to the doctor] and you just get a pill or you get a diagnosis, and that's kind of it. [With PT], you get to form a relationship and really help someone improve their life." Still, Tarr's research on the Alexander Technique—a treatment for back pain that has received little acceptance within scientific communities—has demonstrated how a holistic focus on the whole person can also lead to ostracization from biomedical fields. Tarr notes how the Alexander Technique's "emphasis on the self as a substance to be worked on which is not understood in physiological or anatomical terms" is part of what makes it incompatible with biomedical frameworks (262). In a similar way, it is precisely the move away from generalizable diagnosis and prescription that students described which can lead to a devaluing of physical therapy among medical professionals more broadly (Derkatch).

Finally, with rhetorical body work in mind, it is notable that several students compared PT to other health professions favorably because it was less messy or less directly involved with bodily fluids. This was not a dominant strain of feedback in student responses, but it did arise in several conversations. For example, Clara told the story of how her experience shadowing cousins who were nurses dissuaded her from the profession because "I didn't want to deal with some of the fluids and stuff, just some of the gross parts of that job." Of course, it's notable that Clara's comparison was with nursing, which is lower on the professional hierarchy than PT because it requires less schooling and does not involve a doctorate. When comparing their professional demands with those of doctors, PTs were more likely to mention that they did not want the responsibility of a person's life in their hands or the high-stress career path, though blood was a factor. As Sara put it, "I didn't want an emergency situation. [. . .] A little less blood, a little less life threatening."

Thinking back to Wolkowitz's argument that professional status is accrued by distancing oneself from the body and cordoning it off into parts, the distinctions that students make here between how different professions interact with the body is interesting ("Social Relations" 501). Heightened proximity to the body is another facet of physical therapy that threatens to undermine its professional status among biomedical fields, but here students emphasize their distance from bodily fluids in a way that confers status. Overall, their responses to the question about choosing PT as a profession highlighted the contradictions inherent in the field: Was it more or less scientific than other options? Holistic or biomedical? More or less embodied? It is precisely these contradictions that lead to the boundary-work surrounding scientific expertise that I analyze in this chapter.

Bad Provider Stories

Moving away from the origin stories that students told in interviews to my observations of stories circulating in the lab, one category of story that clearly worked to establish professional identity was the "bad" provider story. These stories typically involved providers outside of physical therapy—nurses, doctors, or others—whose negligent care had to be remedied through the interventions of the physical therapist.

For example, a specialized physical therapist who was an expert in needling techniques told students about caring for a patient with a frozen shoulder. He suspected that she had been given a vaccine into her joint space because she had bruising high up on her arm and her shoulder was sore and achy, which prompted her to come to physical therapy. The moral in this case was about students' patient sense when using needling techniques. The instructor reminded them about double palpating to check for muscle while preparing to insert a needle into one of the students' arms to demonstrate the technique. Because the provider was likely a technician and a one-time contact, there was little else the PTs could do to remedy the situation for the patient except to ensure that they were using proper technique themselves. Of course, the story simultaneously acted as an indictment of the negligent provider even as it instructed students on good technique and embodied awareness.

In other instances, the PT was positioned as the one to help patients navigate troublesome medical directives or even to challenge problematic medical care. An assistant instructor told a story about a patient who was overwhelmed by the doctor's instructions to exercise. She talked about using the TENS technique (applying electrodes to stimulate nerves) that students were practicing to help the patient's swollen knee and to take something off her plate. Here, the PT mediates between the patient and other medical providers. By contrast, other bad provider stories also included an element of pushback from the PT to the other provider. For example, right before starting her demonstration of an effleurage technique to move fluid in a patient's leg, an assistant instructor told the students about a patient who had a lot of fluid in her toe because of a brace on her leg that was too tight. The instructor moved the fluid up using effleurage, a type of massage that involves using the palm of the hand to make circular movements along the body, but also noted that she emailed the doctor about the tightness of the brace.

In these provider stories, the underlying message is clear—as providers with much more frequent and holistic patient contact, the PTs can often be positioned as patient advocates. Meanwhile, by highlighting the occasional negligence of other providers, these PT stories also emphasize the expertise and necessity of their discipline, which can serve as a corrective to depersonalized and occasionally substandard medical care. In this way, their stories resemble arguments midwives made for professional independence from doctors and nurses as well (Spoel and James).

Bad Patient Stories

Along with stories about bad providers came numerous stories about bad patients who either openly resisted care or did not follow directives and suffered for it. At times, these stories demonstrated the limitations of the PT's control over patient actions. An assistant instructor told a story about a patient who had been directed not to use heat on an injury but did anyway, leading to a rash that lasted for nearly three weeks. She closed noting that PTs can educate a patient about risks, but they cannot control the patient's actions.

Other bad patient stories specifically emphasized limiting patient access to PT tools since they were likely to misuse them. For example, the needling expert brought up two different patient stories about needle access. The first described a patient who was asking the PT during care where he could buy similar needles, to which the PT insisted patients should not be needling themselves. At the beginning of the story, the PT noted that the patient had a frontal lobe injury that may have been impacting his judgment and thinking. Of course, students are likely to encounter a range of patients with frontal lobe injuries in their future care—stroke victims or patients with brain injuries make up a large percentage of PT patients. This story positions such patients as unpredictable and not to be trusted, likely to attempt to wrest control of physical therapy interventions from the provider at any moment.

The second needling story imparts a similar message. This story the needling expert attributed to his own instructor, showing how provider stories become an intergenerational source of understanding and disciplinary construction within a field (Ivinson and Renold). He described a teenaged patient whose mother requested several needles to bring home and show her husband, who was not able to attend appointments but was curious about the care. The teenaged girl ended up playing with the needles with friends and breaking off a needle in one of the friends' backs. From there, the story progresses with taking the girl to the hospital only to be told that they had to wait for the needle to come out on its own. The moral is the same as the previous story; patients should never be given needles. However, the hidden curriculum of this story also positions young patients as unpredictable and untrustworthy.

Overall, the PT here becomes the guard of materials and expertise that must be protected from an untrained audience who can cause explicit harm. In this way, bad patient stories, like bad provider stories, work to safeguard expertise and emphasize the necessity of the PT's knowledge and training. At the same time, however, they position patients as opponents who are not to be trusted rather than collaborators in care. None of the patients in these stories are granted innate or intuitive knowledge of their embodied experiences. Thus, the narratives reserve patient sense for the purview of trained providers.

Unruly Patient Bodies

The stories I describe above came from visitors to the classroom who were brought in specifically to share their real-world experiences with students. However, the stories that the main instructor, Kevin, told focused primarily on asking students to troubleshoot their approach to a patient in an unexpected bodily encounter. Rather than having a clear moral, Kevin usually concluded these stories with an open question, "What do you do?" and then engaged in some back-and-forth with students describing possible responses, a kind of Socratic dialogue. This troubleshooting conversation seems less important overall, though, than how these stories work to position PTs and patients in relation to one another and each other's bodies.

The first story Kevin told about a bodily patient encounter was about an early moment in his practice as a PT when he came into the room to find his patient fully undressed. He reflected, "I remember probably my second week post-graduation, I walk in—patient comes in for low back pain—and I walk in and she is naked. And I'm like [wide eyes], 'Okay.'" At this point, Kevin turns the scenario around to the class, asking a male student what he would do: "I come in and there's a naked woman [class laughter]. It happens. What do you think?" Kevin offers "keep a straight face," and then the student suggests offering a covering. Kevin agrees and does an impression of looking down while handing the patient a sheet, saying, "Why don't you take this?" He summarizes the response with "Try to be cool."

At work in this story is the negotiation of professional expectations between patient and provider. As an inexperienced PT, Kevin notes how he was not necessarily prepared for the encounter, whereas the patient's unexpected behavior makes it clear that she may not be familiar with the rules of the environment either. For professionals who are working to highlight scientific expertise and knowledge, distancing themselves from sexualization is particularly important (Ottosson; Wainwright et al.). Thus, notable in Kevin's description here is the way he de-escalates the encounter through his own bodily modification—straight face, trying to be cool—and through the covering of the patient's body, distancing himself from nakedness. Of course, the story brings about laughs for the class in part because of its potentially sexual nature. It is noteworthy that this patient is described only as a woman without age or size details, enabling students to envision her as potentially young and attractive, and that the instructor specifically calls on a male student for his response. A number of Kevin's stories walked a line between making it clear that the therapist's role was to desexualize the patient encounter and showing the potential for patients to bring sexual elements into the interaction.

A similar example arose later that same day, when Kevin prefaced another patient story with the opening "Okay, creepy story time" and then noted that this was a story about "the power of touch." After noting that he has very warm hands, he described a patient encounter:

> I had one patient one time, I'm kind of working on her shoulder. She goes, "Ahhh," making these noises. I'm like "Ew!" [jumps back a little bit], but she keeps doing that. And I'm like "Are you okay?!" and she's like, "Oh God, your hands are just so warm; they're just magnificent." I'm like, "Okay." "Oh your hands, your touch, it's better than sex." I'm like, "Okay, that's really creepy now. You don't have to say that."

As with the naked patient story, this story positions the patient as bringing sexual elements into the physical therapy encounter, this time through physical and verbal reactions to the PT's care. Again, the PT de-escalates by reacting first with disgust (jumping back from the patient) and later by discouraging the patient's sexual comments. Kevin summarized the proper response as "I appreciate that." That is, not undermining the patient relationship by criticizing the response or making them feel awkward, but also not encouraging the sexual conversation. Again, the physical therapist is presented as stoic and distanced, or at least as distanced as they can be while immersed in shoulder massage. The therapist's responsibility is to modulate the bodily interaction to preserve professional status, desexualizing the patient's response.

Counter to these stories of desexualizing patients' responses was a story of modulating one's disgust at the offensive patient body. Again, Kevin introduced this story as preparing students for future patient encounters, commenting, "I'm trying to get you guys ready for patient world; it's coming up." Here, he framed the story as focused on smell and launched into a tale of "one of the smelliest patients I ever, ever had was a dude that raised pit bulls." As with the earlier bodily stories, this story elicited laughs from students. Kevin went on to describe a competition where pit bulls pull weights before providing explicit detail on the patient's stench: "He smelled like a combination of pit bull excrement and pit bull pee and pit bull stink and you would walk into the room and it was a wall of stench. How do you deal?" This time, he called on a female student for feedback. In conversation with the class, they brainstormed several coping strategies, mainly to mask the smell: medical masks, essential oils, Vicks, hand sanitizer, and so forth. Again, Kevin highlighted the necessity of physically modulating the PT body through "keep[ing] a straight face." As with the sexual patient stories, it becomes the provider's responsibility to regulate the patient interaction by concealing disgust, a frequent tenet of emotional modulation in Hochschild's research as well (*Managed Heart*).

Overall, patient stories functioned during the PT lab to build in-group identity among physical therapists. Students recognized the dominance of an "origin story" among their cohort, an encounter with a PT that helped bring them into the profession. Meanwhile, it was clear that storytelling within the lab environment had intergenerational components, with providers bringing in stories that they had been told as students that now lived on through their telling. This identity-building served two key purposes. First, it highlighted PTs' professional expertise and status by demonstrating superiority over other professions and over laypeople. In this way, stories emphasized the necessity of the profession and the way that PTs' scientific training separated them from their patients and other providers, who could not handle a needle properly, as one example.

Notably, in highlighting the PT's embodied expertise, instructors did not account for the patient's embodied knowledge. That is, what innate or intuitive knowledge of their own bodies did patients bring to the encounter, and how might that help to inform a practitioner's care? As Allen points out in her research on individuals with chronic illness, "Just as the EMTs and nurses [. . .]—or Sauer's miners with their 'pit sense'—chronically ill individuals develop intuitive awareness of their bodies' functions and sensations over time. This deep awareness then creates opportunities for patients to notice when something is amiss" (117–18). Part of what distinguishes physical therapy from biomedical professions is practitioners' ability to individualize their care. However, providing personalized care in a responsive way means taking seriously patients' embodied knowledge about their needs and experiences.

Second, patient stories emphasized the physical boundaries between PT providers and patients in line with research in body work, offering students an opportunity to discuss the navigation of these boundaries in fringe cases with their instructor. Often in these cases, the patient is pushing boundaries through sexualization or an unruly body. The instructor and students had opportunities to identify together strategies for both physical modulation (hand them a towel, avert your eyes) and emotional modulation (keep a neutral face) in response to patient actions. In the next section, I consider the physical lessons of the PT lab alongside these narrative lessons.

Body Work in the Physical Technologies Lab

Ultimately, the physical learning that students are practicing in the physical technologies lab marks the beginning of acquiring the bodily comportment of a physical therapist, a process that will continue through their other labs, through clinical placements, and ultimately into their careers. In their research on physiotherapy students, Norris and Wainwright describe a three-part acquisition process during which students are first preoccupied with personal body control, "breaching lines of intimacy and managing social space" (97); then develop concern with interaction through touch; and eventually recognize the communicative potential of touch during clinical placements.

While the physical technologies lab primarily focused on technologies beyond their own bodies, both Kevin and the students were aware that body-to-body care would be their primary intervention with patients in the future. In fact, Kevin framed the goal of many of the technologies as heating up the patient's body so that it would be more mobile for body-to-body intervention. One of his daily mantras during the class was "Warm them up and then do something with them!" He lamented how ineffective physical therapists—and this was often attributed to those in PT chain locations—would use a heat intervention like a heat pack and then just leave the patient immobile, thereby wasting the warming effect.

This section examines both verbal and embodied body-work lessons in the physical technology lab. First, I consider how students were acquiring the patient sense to guide body-on-body contact like massage, demonstrating how they learn this skill in collaboration with their in-class partners and through a process of repeated movement and verbal exchange. Then, I examine lessons in body work at the technology interface, as students acquire embodied practices alongside technological tools like ultrasound wands and electrical stimulation. Given the focus of the labs, technological tools dominated many of the practice sessions I observed, though they were sometimes leveraged more to support understanding of muscle movement and reaction rather than as practice with a tool that students would use on the job.

Learning the Physical Moves

Reflecting on her experience practicing deep tissue massage with her partner, Talia identifies some of the key challenges of learning physical movement techniques in the lab, or really in any professional context that centers body-on-body interaction:

> I didn't know if I was going deep enough, like was I applying enough pressure? So, I think at one point I was asking my partner if the pressure was enough or if it was too much. So, I was definitely learning and getting used to having my hands on somebody and applying pressure. But it was a little hard to know if I was doing it right and I feel like it's hard.

The learning is twofold: understanding what she should be feeling, touching, and manipulating on her partner's body while learning how she should move her own body in response. This requires direct verbal feedback from her partner about their experience of the touch ("was I applying enough pressure?"), but Talia is also wary of constantly eliciting that feedback. Thus, she reflects on wondering much of the time "if I was doing it right," an experience that many of the students shared, especially during lab activities that were focused exclusively on body-to-body contact without other technologies. In this open admission of uncertainty, the development of patient sense is visible. Over time, Talia will just know whether her technique feels right based on the innate knowledge she builds through frequent embodied interactions.

Of course, while learning to move like a physical therapist, students were also learning to verbally interact with future patients by practicing conversation. This included warning the patient about physical touch and requesting their feedback on its intensity but also maintaining small talk even while bridging traditional boundaries between bodies. The degree to which students would use the lab as an opportunity to practice these verbal exchanges varied greatly, often depending on how well students knew one another.

Overall, navigating the complex interplay of physical contact and talk with a near-stranger will be a core tenet in the work of these future physical therapists. This is a challenging type of body work that requires maintenance of physical, emotional, and discursive elements all at once, as students must not just maintain composure but also hold a casual conversation while violating traditional physical boundaries. The ability to do so constitutes professionalism in the field and thus novice physical therapists need opportunities to practice all three elements of bodily comport.

In this section, I consider two physical practice sessions and students' reflections on them when I showed them a clip of their practice during their second interview. I analyze how acquisition of patient sense works alongside verbal learning in the lab context. Both examples are drawn from the beginning of the second week of the lab when students were learning effleurage techniques, a massage that uses the palm of the hand to make circular movements along the body. This section of the lab was directive, as Kevin or his assistant would lead students through effleurage on different areas of the leg.

Getting to Know You

One thing that Kevin highlighted at the beginning of the course was that students were going to be moving away from the small groups they had been using consistently up until that point and would be switching partners and rotating through different classmates.[5] Kevin's lab was the first time these students were all in a room together, and he explicitly encouraged them to change up their partners and work with classmates they did not know as well. At times, like on the day that they practiced effleurage techniques, he would ask students to move to the patient to their left after a practice session to ensure that they worked on someone new.

However, when Kevin did not make these kinds of interventions, students tended to stick to the same small group of friends. As I mentioned above, this impacted students' willingness to practice small talk during their care. In fact, Talia reflected while watching the recording of herself during effleurage practice that her relationship with the other student made her less likely to engage in small talk: "We're friends outside of class, so maybe it's just that we don't have a lot of small talk to make. I feel like with a patient, maybe, that would have been different. But I feel like I could have engaged with the patient

---

5. This was particularly notable because I conducted research during summer 2021, so this was a class that had been impacted by COVID-19 restrictions more than any other and had been kept in small working groups specifically to limit exposure.

a little bit more." Practicing conversational moves while engaging in physical contact came more naturally, then, when students did not have a pre-existing relationship with one another and had genuine information to gather during their care.

This was the case for Bea and Deborah, who were negotiating their previous knowledge of one another while Bea practiced effleurage on Deborah's leg. Bea initially thought that she knew Deborah from high school, but after some back-and-forth, they figured out that Deborah was a year ahead of Bea because she had transferred into the program rather than entering through direct admittance. This conversation was interspersed with frequent checking in about how the effleurage felt, especially as Bea followed new directives from the instructor. Thus, it mirrored the multiple components of body work—physical, verbal, and emotional—that students would engage in with their patients in the future, moving between casual conversation and rapport-building while getting a feel for the kind of physical pressure that is needed and gauging their patient's emotional experience of the care.

Notably, while Bea's lack of familiarity with Deborah supported their verbal exchanges, it also caused her to be more tentative about the amount of pressure she was willing to provide. Bea noted after watching the recording of herself: "You know I'm like testing whether I'm pushing hard enough, I'm not pushing hard enough. I'm asking my partner, 'Oh, is this hard enough or not hard enough?' And then sometimes when she said, 'Oh, it is too hard,' I immediately went back to the nice relaxing one because I was like, 'Oh no, I don't want to hurt her.'" We see Bea's tentativeness here and her retrospective recognition that she might not have been applying enough pressure because she was worried about her partner's reaction. This was something Kevin emphasized frequently to students as well; they were going to have to get used to causing their patients some discomfort, since techniques like effleurage would not be successful if they did not apply enough pressure to the muscles. As they graduated to more openly painful interventions, the group became more used to inflicting a tolerable level of pain on one another. Still, this was always easier to do with someone who was a close friend.

In Bea's case, when she finally did discover a knot in Deborah's leg and dug into it, causing the leg to spasm, the two of them broke down into giggles. In that moment, the nervous energy caused by boundary-breaking physical contact with an unfamiliar partner combined with the sharp physical reaction caused the provider–patient rapport that the two had been practicing to break down. After all, cracking up at a new patient's involuntary physical reaction would be problematic in a real care setting. At the same time, in this moment the women's relationship has graduated from strangers to acquaintances, with the shared laughter supporting the classmate relationship between the two even as it undermines the authenticity of the exchange. In line with my discussion in chapter 2, this echoes both Magelssen's and Singer's arguments about the role that laughter plays in simulation contexts to build in-group identity and comradery.

Crossing Bodily Boundaries

When Kyle was told to switch partners and ultimately found himself practicing effleurage on Bea's back, he faced two challenges: first, he had been the model student for the technique and had not been able to watch Kevin perform it, and second, he had not spent any time practicing care on women, since his previous working group had been all men. Setting up Bea for the massage, he struggled with figuring out how to position a towel over her shorts like Kevin had done during the demonstration. Ultimately, he asked a neighboring student to show him the technique.

This ability to draw on partners or neighboring pairs for information about a technique was also a common strategy among students. For example, later in the semester when Bella was practicing techniques for moving fluid in the leg of a patient with lymphedema, she looked around at her other classmates, trying to get a sense of their movements as she massaged. Ultimately, her partner also intervened to help redirect the massage. Watching herself later, Bella noted, "I remember I struggled with the circular motions because I think I was going in opposite directions at first and so that's when [my partner], she put her hands up like this. I think that was her being like, 'They need to go in the same direction.'" Because of the collaborative space of the lab, with many students all repeating movements together, this physical learning can be easily shared and transferred between students.

However, some techniques—like massaging around a sports bra—could only be acquired through firsthand practice. When Kyle found himself trying to effleurage Bea's back with a sports bra in the way, he struggled to follow the instructor's prompts and navigate the bra. Watching himself later, he reflected on the challenge of maneuvering around the bra when he had only seen the technique performed on men: "[Kevin] went from doing it on a man who's not wearing a bra. Then I went straight away to a woman with one, and I didn't want to be uncomfortable." Kyle reiterated several times while watching his clip that he looked uncomfortable, but he also said that he remembered feeling a bit confused and unsure about how to do the technique but not necessarily uncomfortable. He checked in with Bea frequently about her experience, receiving positive affirmation each time that she was comfortable with the massage.

During her interview, Bea also reflected on the experience and her initial surprise that Kyle was so unfamiliar with navigating a sports bra: "I actually learned a lot the other week when I was paired up with one of the men in our class because it was the first day that we were doing massage and we're working on everybody's backs and he was like, 'I don't know what to do with the fact that you have a sports bra on' because he's only been paired up with other men in the class." The exchange that Bea recounts here demonstrates how switching partners provided students an opportunity not only to practice care on a different type of body but also to encounter how their classmates handled new body types for the first time. Bea is enthusiastic and supportive of Kyle's new experience, even as she reflects on the fact that she had *only* been working with female partners and thus navigating a sports bra was second nature to her. In this case, the lesson about rhetorical body work is less about her own embodied practices and more about understanding how others' physical experiences might be different from her own—how movements and negotiations that come naturally to her might require a lot of thought and physical control for a different classmate.

At the same time, what neither Bea nor Kyle acknowledges explicitly in their reflections on the experience are the bodily boundaries that are being broken when a man is reaching underneath a woman's sports bra like this massage required. Kyle's awkwardness is likely not just a response to the technical difficulty of navigating the bra—as both he and Bea noted—but also to the breaking of these personal boundaries. In addition, his insistence that he did not *feel* uncomfortable, even though he admits while rewatching the clip that he looks uncomfortable, is likely tied to this boundary breaking as well. Since sexual experience and familiarity with women's bodies are often primary tenets of masculine identity, admitting discomfort in this moment has the potential to undermine Kyle's masculinity as well as his still-in-formation identity as a physical therapist. Thus, he identifies the experience as challenging because he was the model for the massage and because he has not massaged over a sports bra before. However, his conscientious checking in with Bea about her comfort level and his hesitance suggest that the sexual nature of the care may also be a contributing factor.

Norris and Wainwright note a similar phenomenon in their research on physiotherapy students, observing, "levels of concern particularly in relation to intimate and sexualized spaces demonstrated different levels of jeopardy. This was in part influenced by past experience but also the gendered and sexed bodies" (97). In their research, concern around entering sexual spaces was particularly visible as students learned and practiced techniques for massaging the pubic area. And as they note, the experience was different for men and women and varied depending on whether they shared the gender of their partner or not, just as Bea's reflection demonstrates.

For all of the students involved, though, the pubic massage became an opportunity to "smack right through" social barriers, which helped students to experience less hesitancy going forward. Norris and Wainwright are skeptical about the efficacy of this approach, noting that it allows students to move beyond social discomfort related to entering sexual spaces and is thus a kind of rite of passage. However, "it potentially condones an approach at odds with the concerns of individual dignity and negotiated acceptability emphasized and expected later" (97). Their conclusion calls for more attention to learning touch as not just a social skill but also a "complex social encounter" (99). After all, even if students become more accustomed to overcoming embodied barriers, that does not mean that their patients will be prepared for these violations of bodily norms. It will be their responsibility to prepare unfamiliar patients for the encounter and to mediate it through regular checks and communication.

The lab offers an opportunity to practice this emotional and verbal body work, though the opportunity can be limited by the fact that students tend to partner with and practice their care on friends and familiars. Kevin's instinct to push students beyond these comfortable circles paid off with opportunities to more thoroughly engage in the small talk of patient conversation and to experience new kinds of physical challenges. While not quite the same as a pubic massage, massaging under a bra necessitated that Kyle "smack through" personal bodily boundaries, which will likely give him more confidence and composure encountering female patients in the future.

Learning the Technology

The majority of lab sessions that I observed (twenty-one out of thirty) included an opportunity for physical therapy students to practice, with one another, using and receiving a technology of some kind. Students spoke of the importance of understanding how interventions felt and passing that knowledge to patients. As Deborah reflected: "I at least want to know what it feels like so I can describe that to my patient." Physical experience with the technologies, then, facilitated verbal patient interactions, providing the means for students to clearly articulate the experience of a technology and help patients to anticipate it. This became particularly important in cases where the intervention might cause pain. Cameron likened this to the way that police officers are tased during training so that they will know what it feels like before tasing someone: "For safety too, so you can let the patient know what they're supposed to feel, so that if they feel something completely different then you can try to fix the problems." Understanding their own pain thresholds, and how experiences of pain and discomfort varied across individuals, was especially important, as I discuss below.

At the same time, Kevin and the students were aware that they would not use these technologies regularly with patients in practice. Many of the electrical stimulation technologies mainly taught students how to recognize and activate different muscles. In this way, technological interactions played a similar role to students' physical experiences of dissection that Fountain discusses. Fountain argues that the objects in his study, including patient bodies, play a key part in constructing the body of the professional: "objects, bodies, and discourses together generate a professional (in this case, medical) subjectivity that emerges in practice and is rooted in bodily activities" (14–15). As students look at diagrams of a hand and then apply motor stimulation to different spots on their partner's hand, watching it contract dramatically and giggling as a group, their embodied learning of anatomy is made visible. Fountain also sees these affordances as socially situated and enacted within the culture of the discipline, highlighting the social and cultural forces that shape enactments.

In this section, I consider two examples of technological learning—one with an ultrasound machine that might be used in PT practice and the other with muscle stimulation that is focused primarily on better understanding anatomy and individual pain thresholds. The lessons in rhetorical body work are more straightforward in the first example, as students practice physically navigating an ultrasound wand on a patient's skin. This is an embodied interaction that will translate directly to clinical practice and which lends students professional expertise specifically through technological know-how. In the second example, lessons in body work are less directly transferable but just as prominent: How does activating different muscles cause different physical reactions? How will a patient respond to pain? How will the students react to a patient's pain response? Part of the hidden curriculum of the lab is tied to how these less directly transferable lessons in body work constitute the field's professional ethos.

New Technologies Promote Attention

As previously described, the interpersonal dynamics between students could really change the degree to which they used lab time to practice patient engagement or to have conversations with friends. Simon and Lauren were close friends, and the beginning of their ultrasound practice session began with amicable chatting. The pair of students next to them was also involved, with the three girls asking Simon if he had had a good nap during the lunch break and telling him what he had missed. Simon was the one delivering the ultrasound care to Lauren's arm, so all of this occurred while he prepared her arm by applying gel and then began adjusting settings on the ultrasound machine, finally using the head of the ultrasound to gently circle the spot on her arm. Lauren teasingly jerked her body at the first touch of the ultrasound wand, pretending it had delivered pain or shock and then burst into giggles. Simon, reflecting on the moment in his interview, rolled his eyes and laughed: "She did that every time."

However, as Simon began delivering care with the ultrasound wand, his attention shifted more fully to Lauren and her physical reactions. Lauren and the pair next to her continued to chat, but Simon was disengaged from the conversation, giving short answers if he responded at all. Watching back a recording of the care, Simon noted this shift as well:

> While I was spreading out the gel before I turn the machine on, I was chatting with everybody beforehand. But as soon as I turn the machine on, I realized I'm very focused in on [Lauren] more so, and people were still talking to me, but I was giving shorter answers and [. . .] I wasn't looking up and talking to them as much. [. . .] I made sure, I guess, that I was looking at her face and I was looking at her when I was doing it and talking to her.

In this way, the new technology shifted Simon's attention to care and especially to attunement with Lauren's physical reactions to the ultrasound. He mentioned specifically looking at her face, which several students referenced as a site for noting if their partners were in pain and gathering nonverbal cues. Being able to deduce physical experience of a technological intervention through facial cues is thus another mode of patient sense that therapists are developing in the lab. While this shift in attention could happen with body-to-body interventions as well, students were more cautious and more attentive when it came to new technologies, recognizing that the capacity for harm was greater and also simply needing to pay attention to a number of different physical moves at once. This resonates with my discussion in the previous chapter of how technologies can productively disrupt and redirect one's attention.

Few of the technologies that students worked with in the lab were complex. The hardest part of many of them was understanding the user interface and how to adjust settings. And yet, adding in a technological component of care necessitated that students navigate even more physical demands. Watching herself perform ultrasound on the back of her partner's leg, Madison explained:

> It looks a lot easier than it is, and it's not hard, but you have to make sure you're keeping an eye on the patient, their verbal and nonverbal cues on how they're doing. Are they feeling gentle warmth? Or if their skin is burning up. Still moving the applicator at a nice slow pace and [covering] the right size of the treatment area so you're not burning them, or so you get an effective treatment. And then keeping the gel where it's supposed to be. And then managing the machine. So lots of little pieces go into it, so just being aware of all those things while you're doing it.

Madison's discussion of the multiple tiers of awareness that are involved in care helps explain Simon's shift in attention as well. While the visible body work of delivering ultrasound care seems straightforward—students are slowly circling an ultrasound head on an exposed area of skin—beneath that action there is a range of mental demands related to bodily comportment and interpersonal engagement. That is, the body work required to navigate this technology effectively is anything but simple, requiring a complex combination of patient sense, interpretation of embodied cues, and verbal patient communication.

New Technologies Highlight Bodily Difference

Part of the reason students had to pay close attention as they applied a technology to their partner in the lab was because their partner's reactions could vary widely. This is what made Lauren's jumping reaction to the ultrasound particularly cruel yet effective—students were always on high alert about causing their partner pain or discomfort. While they could certainly cause harm with body-to-body interactions like effleurage, adding a technology to the scene heightened the risk that their partner would experience something unexpected and painful.

Meanwhile, students noted the wide range of reactions they all had to the different technologies. For example, reflecting on her partner's experience with a neck stabilizer meant to release tension in the head, Isa noted that her partner had experienced release while she had not: "'I feel, like, lighter on my neck area,' is how she described it, because that was something I did end up asking her. I was like, 'Okay, well you said it feels good. What do you mean? What does it feel like?' Because I just thought it [felt] so weird, right? And you want to be able to potentially tell someone, 'This is what you should be looking for.'" Here, Isa describes prompting her partner for more details about her experience with the neck stabilizer so that she would be able to describe it to a patient in the future. Thus, different reactions to the technologies offered students a range of perspectives on potential physical experiences that they could carry with them as providers into future care.

One of the ongoing jokes in the lab occurred when male students, who were often large, former athletes, had low pain tolerance in comparison to others. This was the case for Timmy, whose reaction to receiving electrical stimulation in his arm was notably dramatic. While his group upped the stimulation, Timmy would laugh nervously, grab his arm, and quickly start saying, "Okay, okay," encouraging group members to stop. Walking by, Kevin teased him, "Did you wimp out already? That's going to have to improve." Later, when groups shared out how many milliamps they were able to tolerate during the treatment, Timmy was shocked that he was only at 9 out of 20, when other groups (including the pair of girls next to him) were at 11.

Watching his reaction to stimulation during his interview, Timmy noted: "I remember [the stimulation] would always make me start to panic, like sweating a little bit. I would always laugh, so I know that I saw myself laughing a couple of times, so it's more I need to get better at not laughing." Of course, Timmy would not be the one receiving the treatment in his future work, so getting his laughter under control is less of a priority than being able to describe for future patients what the stimulation might feel like. Still, Timmy's reflection on his laughter demonstrates how controlling emotional responses and having high pain tolerance were tied to the rhetorical body work of physical therapy.

Importantly, because this was a technology that was more focused on learning anatomy than it was on treatment, Timmy's inability to withstand high intensity is more a point of pride than anything else. Several of the male students distinguished themselves from their partners based on their tolerance for high-intensity electrical stimulation. Cameron, who was on the track team, explained how he had had several interventions, including a combination of dry needling with electrical stimulation, which he described as "probably one of the worst things I've ever done." He noted how his partner had asked him to hold off on cranking up the intensity when they were working on shoulder raises with electrical stimulation, "Whereas for me, you know, you could crank it up to full and it would hurt and I wouldn't be comfortable, but I could take it." Similarly, Timmy's partner Robert could not help but compare his own pain tolerance with Timmy's threshold of 9 milliamps during his interview, noting how "after this one we did myself and I got pretty up there. Like the 17 or 18s and I was still feeling fine with it."

One important lesson in body work here is that making assumptions about pain tolerance and embodied experiences based on an individual's appearance is likely misguided. Certainly, several students were inspired by their partner's reactions to treatment to think about how they might frame care for a future patient. For example, Timmy's partner Robert reflected on his experience giving the stimulation, saying:

> I do remember at the time with [Timmy] struggling with the stimulation a bit, trying to justify in my head how would I explain this to a patient if they were having this adverse reaction, that this is beneficial towards them. Because I certainly saw it was something he didn't like and a new sensation that was scary to him and so to try and think about how I would communicate: "This is something that we do in order to elicit a contraction out of you. To get that response from your muscle. And this is a healthy thing, you know."

Thus, from the perspective of professional development, experiencing different pain thresholds and reactions from fellow students provided an important reminder of how to attune to difference in their future body-work practices and to tailor communication for different thresholds.

However, this important learning about embodied difference existed in tandem with a bodily lesson that high pain tolerance was affiliated with masculinity and subsequently also professionalism, which Kevin reinforced with his light teasing of Timmy. When Timmy notes his own need to "get better at not laughing," he is really describing a need for emotional modulation in the face of physical discomfort. This demonstrates the way that pain tolerance and, subsequently, masculinity can become conflated with professionalism within the field of physical therapy. It offers an example of the kind of entrenched masculine values that Frost discusses in her theorization of apparent feminism. Frost argues that especially in technical contexts, political forces have "render[ed] misogyny unapparent at the nexus of social, ethical, political, and practical technical communication domains" (5) and that there is an urgent need to both identify and critique these dominant masculinist perspectives.

In the case of the physical therapy lab, the unexpected reactions to stimulation challenged students' assumptions about bodies. However, the way those heightened reactions from males became the butt of jokes countered potentially productive learning. In this case, while laughter reinforced comradery among students like Magelssen suggests, it also reinforced stereotypes about masculinity and professionalism that are part of the field's hidden curriculum, as Singer similarly finds in his research on trans embodiment in simulations.

In his research on embodied learning in a dissection lab, Fountain talks about objects in the dissection lab offering affordances for disciplinary learning and action, saying: "we enact an object's information through our physical, embodied interaction with that object's affordances, which are opportunities for action that emerge from the mutual contact between the object-ness of the object and our bodily capacities for perception, movement, interpretation, and meaning making" (92). In a similar way, the new technologies in the physical therapy lab could act as a catalyst for student attention and engagement, bringing students into the moment and creating a focus on their partner's reactions, enabling them to also practice patient–practitioner engagement and develop the beginnings of patient sense. Practicing care at the technology interface necessitated focused attention, taking students out of the casual interpersonal relationships that might otherwise dominate their practice. Meanwhile, differing student reactions to and experiences of the new technologies supported students in countering their assumptions about particular kinds of bodies and in considering how to tailor their care for a wide range of needs. Thus, technologies in the lab offered "opportunities for action" both in physical practice of patient care and in linguistic framing of difference.

Hidden Curriculum in the Physical Technologies Lab

Overall, this chapter has demonstrated how the lessons in body work that PT students receive in the physical technologies lab are part of a process of acquiring professional identity in the field. This acquisition process reinforces boundary-work in the PT field, distinguishing it as a unique biomedical discipline with its own scientific knowledge domain. Particularly because professions that center body-on-body contact are at risk of professional denigration, the stories that circulate and embodied practices that are acquired in the PT lab counter the feminized, sexualized, and nonexpert status of body work both explicitly and implicitly. However, in this effort to assert professional status, students also run the risk of acquiring problematic stereotypes about patients and themselves that could undermine the patient–provider relationship.

First, because stories in the lab happen in an ad hoc way, it could be easy to overlook them as a site of critical engagement or revision. However, it is precisely these moments of hidden curriculum that offer possibilities for crucial changes in the perspectives of future providers. In a similar way, we can see how narratives that are designed to reinforce PT's necessity and importance as a field could subsequently lead to unintended consequences—undermining interprofessional collaboration or setting up mistrustful patient relationships. The presentation of patients as at times deceitful and certainly misguided in understanding their own needs directly contradicts the larger ethos in holistic health fields to trust and rely upon patient's embodied knowledge. While patient and provider stories serve necessary in-group functions, I am also wary of the ways that they position other patients and providers that potentially reinforce stereotypes and could lead to worse outcomes for specific groups. That makes attending to these narratives all the more important. In line with body work, it is also notable how the narratives of the PT lab are often created in reaction to the central role of body work within the profession, to counter the denigrating effects that regular contact with the body can create for a field.

In addition, while the body-on-body learning in the lab highlights the possibility of bodily variation among their patients, students are also limited by the variety of bodies that are available among a population of young, healthy graduate students. Reflecting on her experience practicing moving fluid in the leg of a patient with lymphedema, Bella noted: "It's hard to get a feel because they don't have fluid in their legs. I don't know what it would feel like if you actually [. . .] had lymphedema that you were trying to move." Thus, while other students' bodies offer more authentic physical experiences than the patient manikin in chapter 2, they still cannot represent even close to the spectrum of physical encounters students will have in the future. The group is, by and large, much more fit and physically able than their future patients will be, making it difficult to approximate much of the movement and patient sense they will need to acquire.

Finally, in students' interfaces with technology in the lab, we can see how the specific social and cultural context of the discipline brackets the potential for learning about physical variation as well. By conflating pain tolerance with both masculinity and professionalism, students learn that their own physical reactions must be modulated and contained, a tenet of much training in body work. Meanwhile, stereotypes about men and their relationship to pain are reinforced, shaping the way that future providers will approach their care of different bodies, both feminine and masculine. In their research on students in a massage program, Wainwright et al. note how "the encouragement to perform a less stereotypical embodiment of femininity or defeminisation is justified primarily on the grounds of health and safety and professionalisation. [. . .] But it is also implicitly linked to the purposeful desexualisation of the environment" (84). Similarly, we can see how efforts to desexualize PT practice through masculinization might have unintended consequences as well.

As with the patient debriefs in nursing simulations, PT students will benefit from constellating possibilities rather than defaulting to narrowly defined roles and responses. This suggests the value of bringing in a range of positions and perspectives to both in-class narratives and embodied exchanges to ask how students might change their care in response (Campbell, "Simulating Gender"). Much of this practice will have to be imagined (i.e., "What modifications would you make to that technique for a patient who is obese / does not have motor control of their femur / has recently suffered a stroke?"). Still, similar questions would push students to think beyond the narrow graduate student population that is their focus. The physical technologies lab was already engaged in a dialogic approach to discussing patient stories and practicing patient care, where students and instructor would brainstorm possibilities for action together. Thus, constellating possibilities for different patient bodies and experiences in conversation would be a natural fit.

Also, in line with Press's argument that medical simulations should include perspectives from marginalized groups, the lab would benefit from increased feedback from both marginalized providers and patients to ensure that individuals from a range of diverse backgrounds are actively involved in telling stories and practicing embodied exchange. While Kevin brought in assistants and guests to speak to niche areas of professional expertise, there is also a possibility to consider what kinds of demographic perspectives these individuals can offer in expanding students' perspectives of their future patients.

This chapter demonstrates how the framework of rhetorical body work brings a new dimension to our understanding of scientific boundary-work. While Gieryn initially positioned boundary-work as rhetorical, he focused primarily on stylistic resources including literary devices like metaphor, hyperbole, and antithesis (781). Contemporary rhetorical research on boundary-work has expanded its purview significantly but also maintained a textual focus. For example, authors focus on the discursive work scientists do to assert professional status in arenas like professional journals (Bazerman; Derkatch), accreditation documents (Spoel and James), and interprofessional tools like knowledge maps (Wilson and Herndl).

However, rhetorical body work is vital to understanding scientific boundary-work for two reasons. First, because frequent body-on-body contact has the potential to undermine professional status and scientific expertise, relegating touch professions to the realm of CAM. Therefore, fields that frequently engage in body work and rely on difficult-to-quantify patient sense are inherently tied up in boundary-work to counter professional denigration. And second, because boundary-work is embodied in addition to discursive, constituting a way of movement and physical interaction that emphasizes scientific knowledge and expertise, often through a process of defeminization and desexualization.

This embodied boundary-work is necessary for fields that are working to maintain professional status and recognition like physical therapy. Yet this chapter also demonstrates the potentially negative consequences in students' understanding of themselves as providers and their patient sense that accrue because of embodied boundary-work. By constellating possibilities for bodies within the lab, instructors can work to counter some of these problematic assumptions. It is also worth noting that the masculine logics that dominated the space contributed to the potentially problematic physical lessons. Resonating with Frost's theory of apparent feminism that posits that misogynistic perspectives are often normalized and invisible within technical domains, my findings demonstrate how fields aspiring to accrue or maintain scientific status can often be drawn into masculinist cultural logics like efficiency and rationality. By emphasizing masculine values, practitioners can subsequently devalue patient sense, which fields like physical therapy and midwifery often use to distinguish themselves from more mainstream biomedical professions (Spoel and James). Toeing the line between individualized and responsive care and scientific status, then, remains an ongoing challenge for the touch professions.

CHAPTER 4

Reaching through the Screen
Mediated Body Work in a Virtual Intensive Care Unit

The virtual intensive care unit (VICU) is always bustling, but the bustle is different from what you might experience on a hospital floor. A nurse is walking over to check in with another nurse about something she has seen in a patient chart; a nurse practitioner is on the phone with a patient asking about their breathing; a tele-observer is speaking over her microphone into a patient's room, reminding them to stay in their bed. All the care is mediated—through phones and computer screens, microphones and video cameras. And yet, the room also ebbs and flows with the cadence of a hospital day—more back-and-forth questioning during check-ins with the floor nurses, more patient directives from the tele-observers in the evening when the patients under surveillance do not have family or providers around to distract them.

This chapter focuses on the tele-observers in the VICU, specifically how they practice body work in their day-to-day interactions with patients and other providers and rely on patient sense to support their decision-making. Tele-observers virtually monitor high-need hospital patients through video cameras in the patient's room, typically observing six to eight patients at a time and communicating with them using a microphone. Their role has replaced what used to be called patient sitting, where one hired individual would stay in the room with a high-risk patient 24/7 to monitor their actions. To do this job virtually, tele-observers draw on a diverse knowledge base of prior experiences and on their emplacement in the VICU space to inform their choices and shape their practice.

In the VICU, each tele-observer is positioned in front of a dual-monitor screen featuring six to eight small video feeds of patients in their hospital rooms. Tele-ops[1] can click into each feed and see an enlarged view of the patient as well as hear sound in the patient's room. Their job is to make sure that patients are not violating protocol by getting out of bed or otherwise disturbing their IV lines, oxygen tubes, or other medical interventions. If protocol is broken, tele-observers are responsible for issuing a "redirect," either by speaking verbally into a microphone connected to the room or pushing a button that delivers an automated verbal command. If a patient does not respond to their redirect, the tele-observer may call a nurse or sound a stat alarm,[2] depending on the situation's severity. Tele-observers also have a set of paper documents where they keep track of how often patients break protocol and their interventions. Tele-ops share the VICU room with virtual nurses and nurse practitioners, who have separate responsibilities for remote patient care but are sometimes leveraged in the decision-making process, as I describe later.

As tele-ops navigated this complex set of mediated patient observations and interventions, they drew on prior workplace experiences to make strategic choices about when and how to intervene with patients and other providers. Unlike the students in chapters 2 and 3, tele-observers did not come to this work through a sequenced curriculum designed to prepare them for professional practice. While certified nursing assistant (CNA) certification was recommended for the position,[3] not all tele-observers had that training. Instead of, or in addition to formalized training, they drew on professional experiences in a wide range of fields, some closely tied to healthcare like being a lab technician in an oncology unit, and others far afield, like working in airline customer service and owning a coffee shop. Drawing on this wide range of experiences, tele-ops attentively read physical cues on their screens, drawing on patient sense to make choices about whether to intervene, as well as choices about adjusting their own tone and volume. Meanwhile, they modulated their emotions and those of their collaborators, often navigating mistrust from nurses who expect them to catch every patient mishap. Overall, tele-ops are constantly enacting complex embodied communication strategies and

---

1. Tele-observers were also frequently referred to as "tele-operators" in the VICU, or "tele-ops" for short.

2. The stat alarm is a loud alert that sounds throughout the hospital floor. In a discussion of alarm fatigue on the AvaSure corporate website, Todd Sloane describes the tele-sitting system's stat alarm as "one alarm you will respond to," citing both its volume and its direct connection to an immediate threat to a patient or provider. He says the average response time by providers to an AvaSure stat alarm is fourteen seconds.

3. To gain this certification, individuals take a two-credit course offered through local community colleges followed by a certification exam (the National Nurse Aide Assessment Program examination).

relying heavily on intuitive knowledge and cues, despite their positioning in a virtual healthcare context.

Based on interviews with seven tele-observation workers and twenty hours of observation in a VICU in the upper Midwest, this chapter unpacks the embodied practices and patient sense that workers from a wide range of professional backgrounds bring to tele-observation. I begin with background on embodiment in virtual care contexts before moving into analysis of different aspects of the tele-op's professional body work. This includes unpacking my participants' professional backgrounds and how their prior work experiences impact their patient sense on the job; discussion of their relationship to and negotiation with patients and other practitioners—especially bedside nurses; and their reflections on the physical experience of the job and its connection to future roles. Across these sections, I reflect on how the virtual context of the VICU transforms rhetorical body work but also reinforces its necessity.

One of the goals of this chapter, then, is to draw on the lens of body work and the concept of patient sense to demonstrate the complex expertise that tele-workers bring to their jobs, expertise that draws on both their professional histories and their emplacement in the shared space of the virtual intensive care unit. As I show, this body work cannot be easily replicated by an algorithm or an international worker thousands of miles away, as it relies on tele-observers' unique patient sense, drawn from prior experience in combination with the specific environmental cues of the VICU. As we prepare students, especially those outside of traditional academic pathways, for work in the rapidly changing field of healthcare technology (van den Broek; Lapum et al.), we have much to learn from practitioners who are always in the process of adapting their prior embodied experiences for new professional contexts.

Embodiment in Virtual Care Contexts

The shifting nature of healthcare delivery has inevitably changed the work of patient care for providers who previously gained knowledge through direct patient contact. While some have argued that this shift to virtual care disembodies the work of providers, many recognize the ongoing need for attention to workers' embodied practices in this virtual space. In the early 1990s, Hayles argued for a materiality of informatics that could account for the "changing habits of posture, eye focus, hand motion, and neural connections that are reconfiguring the human body in conjunction with information technologies" (149). Meanwhile, in their research on virtual collaborations between software teams in India and Dublin, Vidolov and Vidolov demonstrate the role of virtual embodiment between workers which includes co-presencing (mutual visibility), co-orienting (mutual attunement and readiness to engage), and co-investing (mutual attunement of care and commitment). Their research highlights the physical aspects of virtual embodiment, including things like posture and screen visibility to demonstrate engagement, but also emotional components that contribute to a sense of mutual care: "being there for the other or orientated towards one's needs and concerns" (6503).

Similarly, in his research on body work in international call centers in India, Rajan-Rankin emphasizes the numerous ways that "the fleshy body is evoked" both in terms of workers' physical comportment in the call center space, where they are highly monitored for posture and dress, and of workers' emotional comportment over the phone, where they adjust accents and tone to evoke certain identities in the "corporeal imaginaries" of those on the phone line (19). Rajan-Rankin's research calls attention to the racialized dynamics of these virtual interactions as well, where both worker and caller are involved in a complex negotiation of identity performance and interpretation.

Just as providers' embodiment is shifting in virtual workplaces, the bodies of patients are also transformed. As Sandelowski explains in her research on tele-nursing, providers are "no longer simply encountering their patients directly as manifestly physical presences, they now increasingly encounter them indirectly as virtual presences on screen and over telephone lines" (63). How does patient sense transform when it becomes virtual patient presence? Sauer discusses similar questions when she considers the design of robotic sensors to guide human decision-making in the mines. She notes that rather than thinking of these technologies as a replacement for human senses, "the system must have two-way communication between the human miner and the machine" because the system will never be able to fully capture the amount of sensory information the miner is receiving ("Embodied Knowledge" 161).

Thus, patient sense still exists in the virtual context, as I will demonstrate, though it is mutually informed by the environmental cues that are available through video and audio systems in the VICU, as well as the tele-observers' prior human encounters in different kinds of professional positions. This two-way communication—the incorporation of tele-workers' body work into decision-making with technological systems—is even more important when we recognize the racial and cultural biases that are often embedded in this infrastructure and the ways that it can reinforce existing disparities in healthcare.

The stories of technology failing to achieve equitable outcomes in healthcare are numerous and widespread. Graham outlines several failures of medical technology, including a button for race on incentive spirometers (used to measure lung capacity) that made it more difficult for Black workers to receive workers' compensation (12) and pulse oximeters that were primarily tested on white patients and delayed intervention for Black patients during the COVID-19 pandemic (13). While these limitations may seem to be more about the tools, it is important to remember that a tool's measurements soon become part of black-boxed algorithmic tracking that will ultimately tell a practitioner whether to intervene or alert a provider about a potential problem. Thus, our interfaces are "sites within which the ideological and material legacies of racism, sexism, and colonialism are continuously written and re-written" (Selfe and Selfe 484).

Noble and Benjamin expand on these claims about how algorithms encode racial biases. Noble's work focuses specifically on search engine algorithms, while Benjamin coins the term "the new Jim Code" to describe "the employment of new technologies that reflect and produce existing inequities but that are promoted and perceived as more objective or progressive than the discriminatory systems of a previous era" (5–6). In her book on tele-mental health, Bedor Hiland similarly argues that fetishizing new technologies often distracts designers from addressing systemic barriers in healthcare. In the case of mental healthcare, these technologies are touted for providing access, when they mainly promote convenience for practitioners and patients who would already be using the services. While the use of tele-observation is more widespread across demographic groups, it runs similar risks of being idealized as a money-saving, lifesaving technology while its limitations for both patients and providers are overlooked or ignored.

A Brief History of Tele-Observation

Unlike other virtual healthcare practices, tele-observation, also known as virtual patient monitoring, already experienced significant growth and integration into healthcare prior to the COVID-19 pandemic. Before it was introduced, tele-sitting required that a single observer be physically present in a hospital room with a single high-risk patient 24/7. By contrast, tele-observers can monitor numerous patients at once on video cameras from a remote location with similar—and sometimes even superior—rates of fall prevention (Votruba et al.). Scholars also report the effectiveness of tele-sitting to monitor "safety concerns such as patient elopement, drug use, self-harm, and dislodgement of medical devices" (Sand-Jecklin et al. 146). As such, tele-sitting has become widespread in medical systems nationwide; a prominent TeleSitter system, AvaSys, was being used in over three hundred healthcare facilities as of 2020 (Krasniansky).

However, the movement of healthcare into virtual contexts has the potential to increase professional precarity for providers both because it can transform their work into gig work and because it can lead to the devaluing of their technical knowledge and their embodied expertise. This is particularly salient for my participants because most of them did not have four-year degrees and instead drew on a combination of nursing-assistant training and prior experience to perform their work. While my participants' tele-observer positions had a good deal of stability, the movement of this work into a virtual context has the potential to compound its devaluing. Bedor Hiland describes how this devaluing occurs in the context of tele-mental health providers, who, while they tout the benefits of flexibility and low overhead that accompany the job, also must make themselves available at all hours and rely heavily on clients finding them within a sea of online options. Bedor Hiland also emphasizes how psycho-surveillance—the monitoring of others' mental states online—has now become unpaid, high-risk labor that is expected of good virtual citizens in spaces like Facebook (73).

While it is unlikely that tele-observation would ever become a responsibility of the public,[4] it was clear to me in interviews that the very aspects that make it an appealing job for participants—its limited physical toll and virtual distance from patients—also make it vulnerable to outsourcing or reduced investment. Meanwhile, tele-observers emphasize the importance of having a cohort in a shared space while they work, arguing that doing this deeply emotional work alone would be devastating. Describing her previous experience observing stroke patients alone, one participant noted: "what was the most difficult about that job was that when you have situations that you're watching, you have nobody to talk to about it. And that's so important as a human being, I think, to be able to defuse." Thus, the professional devaluing of telework has potentially wide-reaching consequences for providers, who may find themselves in less stable positions and more isolated if administrators choose to reduce resources.

Overall, tele-sitting aligns with many of the priorities of a neoliberal health system in the United States, reducing costs and increasing provider capacity without sacrificing quality of patient care, and thus it is likely to continue expanding. The remaining question for many is the degree to which AI might take over the role of tele-sitters in the future, automating the job and reducing

---

4. Though, perhaps I should not be so dismissive. The possibility of using volunteers as tele-sitters has certainly been considered. In their review of literature on video monitoring, Davis et al. report that "the use of unpaid adults who volunteered or who were family/friends has been found to be cost effective, however, the reliance of volunteers to staff units around the clock is difficult" (238).

costs even further. This is a possibility that I dispute as I demonstrate the complex contextual and embodied knowledge that tele-sitters leverage on the job every day. Instead, I call for more attention to how we educate tele-sitters of the future, an area that has been so far neglected in favor of ad hoc preparation and training (Sand-Jecklin et al. 148). Given that tele-observers' patient sense emerges at an intersection between prior educational and workplace experiences and their emplacement in the unique environment of the VICU, understanding how to leverage both sources of embodied knowledge in their decision-making is a crucial skill that could be taught.

Field Context

The Virtual Intensive Care Unit

The virtual intensive care unit featured in this chapter is run by a large academic medical hospital network in southeastern Wisconsin. It is located in an office building rather than a clinical one, alongside offices and workspaces for hospital administrators. Virtual nursing and tele-observation staff in the VICU provide remote clinical monitoring 24/7 for hospitalized patients in three different hospital locations. During summer 2021, I conducted approximately twenty hours of observations in the VICU. The following summer, I reached out to the tele-observer team specifically and conducted seven interviews about their experiences via video conference. Since the VICU was the only context that involved real patients, my data collection looked different than at my other two sites. I did not have permission to record live conversations between practitioner and patient and therefore could not video record in the space. Still, I felt fortunate to have access to the space and to observe communication in action.

But how did I find myself in the VICU at all? This story begins with a radio interview that my colleague overheard on a local station while commuting to work. The interview was discussing a new patient-deterioration algorithm—the Rothman Index—being implemented by this hospital network. The interviewee described the algorithm as capturing nurses' intuition and my colleague's ears perked up; she and I had just finished a long-term project studying how provider intuition facilitates patient communication and care (Campbell and Angeli). What would it mean for an algorithm to capture provider intuition? We were suspicious of this claim, but curious.

I will spare some of the details of the winding trajectory that the project took from here. In short, we brought in collaborators from computer science and management while my colleague decided to prioritize other projects. Our team received an NSF pilot grant to study algorithmic decision-making in the VICU, a proposal we submitted in early March of 2020. Naturally, COVID-19 derailed the project in many ways, as the VICU nurses quickly pivoted from remote monitoring of hospital patients to triaging ambulatory COVID-19 patients.[5] By the time we were able to conduct observations on-site during summer 2021, the nurses were primarily focused on offering and booking appointments for monoclonal antibody therapy to COVID-19 patients that qualified. They were also beginning to engage more with remote patient monitoring programs for conditions like mental health and diabetes. Meanwhile, the hospital had ended its contract with the Rothman Index. Thus, my observations and conversations with the VICU nurses bore out some interesting findings about the implementation of algorithms in patient care and the shifting landscape of telemedicine (Campbell et al.). However, I also became increasingly interested in the other group of providers in the room, the tele-observers.

The VICU is an open room with approximately six nurse and nurse practitioner stations spread across one side of the room and approximately eight tele-observation stations on the other side of the room. While all the providers have standing desks, during my observations the nurses were much more likely to have their desks elevated, facilitated by extra space between each of their stations. Tele-observers typically sat close to one another at their dual monitors with headphones on and a double screen featuring video footage of six to eight patients. They would click into different video streams to enlarge them and listen in on the room for a few minutes. Occasionally, I would hear them speaking to patients in the room, asking them to get back into bed: "Mr. Jones, Mr. Jones, what are you doing? Please get back into your bed." While there was more interaction among members of the same team than across the two groups, VICU nurses and tele-observers would occasionally collaborate, especially when technological issues arose or a tele-observer needed to take a break.

My virtual interviews with tele-observers ranged from thirty minutes to one hour in length and included several questions about their professional history and background in addition to information about their day-to-day practices in the VICU (see appendix 3). Since tele-observers were not required to

---

5. An ambulatory patient means literally one who can walk around, but in the VICU this term was used to describe patients with confirmed COVID-19 who were not currently in the hospital. These patients were often monitored remotely by VICU nurses using tools like pulse oximeters to decide whether they would need admittance or readmittance to the hospital and to offer relevant interventions, like monoclonal antibody therapy.

have professional certification (a CNA certificate was preferred) and received little on-the-job training, I was particularly interested in what aspects of their prior experiences were informing their physical and verbal workplace practices. Even though the VICU was not an explicitly pedagogical context like the simulation and physical therapy labs, my questions homed in on the diverse experiential learning that influenced tele-observers' body work on the job. I had a set of questions about previous work and educational experiences, in addition to questions about communication strategies and embodied practices in the VICU.

My Body on the Scene: Power Down

It's 8:30 p.m. on a Thursday evening in early June. I am in the VICU for one of several evening observations, so that I can get a sense of how operations change during the night shift. One of the nurses has alerted me that evening tends to be a busier time for the tele-op team. During the day, patients have doctors, family, meals, and more interaction to keep them preoccupied and following their protocols. In addition, several of the patients will experience sun downer's syndrome, making them more confused and restless in the evenings. This is proving to be true as the tele-ops sound busy, speaking frequently into their microphones to redirect their patients.

There have already been some technical difficulties during this shift with one of the VICU nurses discovering she cannot view the video stream from a camera in a patient's room. She asks another nurse to check the camera, and when they both confirm they cannot see the patient, they call information technologies (IT) support. Several minutes later, however, all the cameras go down so that no one in the room can livestream their patients. Immediately, the providers become frenzied; one of the nurses makes a call to IT while all the tele-ops begin phoning bedside nurses to let them know they are no longer monitoring. What was once a relatively quiet room with periodic directives coming from the tele-ops' side is now filled with a cacophony of noise. While the tele-ops seem to be getting through to their bedside nurses, the nurses are having trouble reaching IT and are scrambling to find a resource book with all the phone numbers.

Eventually, the group concludes that it is the platform that connects patient video cameras to the VICU that has gone down, and some phone calls are not working because they are being routed through that platform. The charge nurse in the VICU manages to get in touch with IT, and one of the other nurses contacts the manager of the VICU to update her on the situation. The group restarts the system, and within the next couple of minutes the cameras are back up and running. However, the crash has called attention to the risks of such a technologically networked system. Not only were tele-ops unable to stream video of their patients, but they also could not reach bedside nurses through the system to notify them about the problem. Luckily, the phones were still working, but otherwise, the bedside team might have been completely unaware of the outage and loss of patient surveillance. Sitting in the room with the team, I could feel the palpable anxiety of an outage like this, where a technological crash means that both patient care and team communication are interrupted.

Employment Experiences and Patient Sense

> Frances worked in banking, then as a CNA and a registered nurse, before quitting to own a coffee shop. Ginny started her career as a CNA and then worked in an oncology unit, first as a receptionist and then as a lab technician. She then spent fourteen years teaching special education before transitioning back into healthcare. Carter described a forty-year-long career in call centers, airline customer service, public schools, and as an investigator of health insurance claims.

The participants I interviewed from the VICU had remarkably diverse professional backgrounds; they also represented a range of ages (twenty to sixty) and racial backgrounds (see table 1). While rhetoric of health and medicine scholarship has been attentive to the embodied experiences of patients as they navigate complex health systems in their day-to-day lives (Kessler; Arduser; Jeffrey Bennett; Swacha), the embodied experiences of providers are less often an area of focus. Meanwhile, the focus remains primarily on providers in professional career tracks, reflecting larger biases in technical and professional writing toward positions that require four-year degrees (Rose) and, especially, medical doctors (Campbell, "Rhetoric of Health" and "Not Just Doctors"). However, as my conversations with the VICU team will demonstrate, tele-observers are leveraging a wide range of prior experiences to inform their embodied practices. These include formal education as well as a wide variety of professional roles.

Drawing on my participants' reflections about connections between their prior experiences and the VICU, this section demonstrates how participants drew on a wide range of embodied knowledge gained through prior experiences to shape their patient sense. As tele-op Carter explained: "You take your experiences in life [. . .] over the time that you've had of just interacting with people on the daily. Just incorporate all of that, whether it's work, personal, or just everything in between. You just try to grab bits and pieces of this and that and try to get through it." "It" includes deep consideration of patients' physical cues, of the impact of different kinds of auditory interventions, of one's own emotional attachment and engagement with individual patients. "It" includes drawing on relational knowledge of individuals with different diagnoses and with nursing staff to contextualize their physical and emotional responses. "It" means a different kind of emotional and physical modulation than what happens on the hospital floor, that makes the virtual job both tenable and meaningful.

In this section, I begin by describing key aspects of the onboarding process for new tele-observers in the VICU, as well as gaps that participants believed existed in the current training. Then, I discuss how participants' prior roles impacted their work practices in their view. Table 1 describes my seven participants and their previous work experiences. I have organized these roles into student, customer service, and other healthcare contexts in my analysis. However, those categories are capacious, with most participants taking on

TABLE 1. Overview of tele-observer study participants

PSEUDONYM	GENDER	RACE	AGE	PART-/FULL-TIME	TIME IN VICU	PREVIOUS WORK EXPERIENCE
Ava	woman	Black	20s	PT	1 year	biology undergraduate student; CNA
Becca	woman	Black & white	30s	PT	4.5 years	CNA; health aide; childcare provider; family care provider; medical aide; social work student
Carter	man	Black	48	FT	1 year	call center employee; airline customer service provider; school paraprofessional; subrogation analyst
Darilyn	woman	Black	40s	PT	2 months	phlebotomist; triage coordinator; CNA
Evie	woman	white	43	FT	5 years	residential caregiver; customer service provider
Frances	woman	white	62	PT	6 months	bank assistant; CNA, registered nurse; coffee shop owner; patient services representative
Ginny	woman	white	50s	PT	2 years	CNA; Oncology receptionist; Oncology lab technician; special education paraprofessional; EEG monitoring technician

roles in all three at some point during their careers, and with many articulating different and, at times, contradictory influences from those roles.

VICU Onboarding

The job ad for tele-op staff in the VICU identifies a preference for individuals with previous clinical or patient care experience as well as accreditation through a paramedic, EMT, CNA, or medical assistant program, "CNA preferred." Five of my seven participants had CNA accreditation, and all of them had some interface with the medical field previously, Carter's being the most tangential as an investigator of health insurance claims. Thus, the onboarding process for the VICU seemed designed with a certain level of existing knowledge about healthcare operations and patient needs in mind. Participants noted that things like medical terminology and hospital operations were necessary for the job, but that they either started with that knowledge or learned it once they started working. Ava mentioned watching a few videos focused on patient care, like common signs of a heart attack, but said that most of these videos seemed created "for the people working in the hospital." Tele-observers were much more likely to be observing patients who were under supervision for self-harm or dementia, making heart attacks unusual, for example.

Thus, when asked about training for the job, most participants described a focus on the technology they would be using, the visual program for video monitoring, and the vocal system that allowed them to use a microphone to speak to patients in the room. Becca explained that their training was "more so of how to navigate the system, the computer system, the screens." Evie described several weeks of onboarding, during which she learned one system and then had time to practice using it alongside a mentor: "There'd be another week of us sitting in the hot seat and just kind of playing around with the screens and zooming in and out on the patient's rooms and pulling up cameras, discharging and admitting patients." Others mentioned admitting and discharging patients from tele-observation as a key component of their early learning as well, focusing both on the logistical side of this process, which differed even across hospitals within the same system, and the reasoning for monitoring.

Ginny, who had spent the previous twelve years working as an electroencephalography (EEG) monitor for patients with seizures on the hospital floor, felt strongly that more contextual knowledge about the hospital and its operations should be incorporated into training. Specifically, she mentioned the need for more attention to when tele-ops use their voice to speak to patients versus when they use an automatic, robotic voice generated by the computer, and when they choose the stat alarm. She noted that these choices were patient-specific: "There are times where people are in mental states where [using the automated voice] would not be a good thing to do," and that training had overemphasized the stat alarm as an intervention, when "I think it can be a negative thing for people." The ability to read physical cues and think about the impact that different tones and sound would have on a patient's body speaks to the counterintuitive way that tele-ops relied on patient sense even in their virtual context. For many, physical experience in hospital contexts played a key role in how they performed their job in the VICU, as I describe below.

Ginny also thought that more emphasis should be put on how to ask the nurses for information to understand patient needs: "Where I notice that people that come into tele-monitoring that haven't had a relationship with [hospital nurses], you almost have to develop that type of trust that you have with that nurse because then you're a team." As I discuss below, several participants noted how their hospital experiences helped them to be better collaborators with the nursing staff on the hospital floor. While this might be hard to teach explicitly, it certainly was a key element of success on the job, and one directly tied to body work since it required modulating their emotions and countering mistrust from nurses who believed they might be slacking off.

Formal Education

While most of my participants had CNA training, most of this training had occurred many years ago. Only Ava, who was currently an undergraduate student studying biology, had received her CNA training recently. Meanwhile, Becca, who was working part-time in tele-ops and part-time as a medical assistant in a family clinic, was earning credits toward a master's degree in social work. Thus, the two of them were able to speak most directly to how their formal education informed their work in the VICU. Mainly, they emphasized how classroom content helped them better understand and empathize with their patients and with other providers because they knew more about certain conditions and different hospital roles.

Ava noted that while she was learning more about different illnesses in CNA training, this information was of limited use because "we can't call the nurse and say, 'hey, the patient is having a seizure.'" Because diagnosis was outside of a tele-op's role—and outside of a nurse's role as well—being able to identify illnesses was not immediately useful. However, her ability to contextualize patient experiences by better understanding how medical diagnoses might be connected to specific behaviors was helpful. When asked how her social work courses influenced her work in tele-ops, Becca reflected on this contextualizing ability: "Understanding why people do the things that [they] do. Commit, or try to commit, suicide. Or the reasons why. It's just so many different forms of mental health out there. I'm really learning the schizophrenic, the narcissist, just the different forms of it. So, I'm kind of seeing how people act it out in the emergency rooms or in the different hospitals." Here, Becca shows how the information she is learning in coursework about different mental health diagnoses informs her interpretation of patient behavior on the screen in tele-ops. These diagnoses are embodied by her patients on the screen as they "act it out," both giving her classroom learning more real-world application and helping her to contextualize the patients she is observing. As she explained later in the interview, since tele-ops do not have access to patients' charts or backgrounds—"we just know that they're [in the intensive care unit] for suicide"—this contextual information about mental health diagnoses is sometimes all she has to help understand patient experience and action. Like the patient preparation sheet in simulations, it becomes a cue for informing tele-ops' patient sense and interventions.

In a similar way, Ava talked about how her coursework as a CNA contributed to her empathy for the patients she was observing. Empathy, she argued, was a big focus in her CNA training, and she was learning to consider the many factors that might lead to a patient acting out: "You don't think about, 'hey they're in a lot of pain, they're under a lot of stress, they might be trying to figure out how they're going to pay for this treatment.'" Here, Ava not only considered how a patient's diagnosis might influence behavior but also how other aspects of their experience might influence their physical actions. Ava's patient knowledge from CNA training, then, encourages her to modulate her own emotions and the patient's by considering those emotions in relation to a challenging set of circumstances—social, physical, and even financial. The students in Britt's research on the legal clinic experience a similar phenomenon when their learning about structural inequities in class is then enacted through their physical and emotional work with vulnerable clients.

Ava also described her CNA training as contributing to her empathy for other providers, especially the nurses on the hospital floor. She described learning to think about the many demands on nurses' time: "I understand the stress that both sides are under so I'm definitely mindful with working virtually [. . .] just being very understanding with the nurses." This was a lesson that those with healthcare experience in other arenas mentioned frequently as well, arguing that they were better able to navigate care alongside a nursing team because of their physical knowledge of what it was like to be on the hospital floor.

Customer Service

Several of my participants had worked in corporate settings in addition to, or in between, stints in healthcare contexts. For example, Evie mentioned that alongside her work in residential care services, she had worked in customer service. She connected the dots between the careers, saying, "I worked with customers a lot. That's my one thing—taking care of people and helping people." Meanwhile, Carter spoke the most about the connections between his corporate work and his work in tele-ops because he had not had direct experience in a healthcare setting. Here, I dig into his discussion about prior work experience and his practices as a tele-op to consider the physical and emotional learning he brought from customer service into virtual patient monitoring. I consider how Carter's patient sense developed out of previous interactions with customers and, thus, shaped his approach to rhetorical body work in the VICU.

Carter's career background included call center work, airline assistance, as well as fifteen years as a paraprofessional in a public school system, and a period analyzing health insurance claims. Like Evie, he drew parallels between these experiences with their outward focus on helping people: "It's a well-rounded thing of interacting with people and assisting, and problem-solving and things of that nature, so just a little bit of everything there." When he was describing his airline work, he even inadvertently drew a parallel to tele-op work by conflating customers and patients: "You're either boarding patients— uh, patients, boarding customers [laughs]—checking them in, taking their bags." The job most directly related to patient care, however, was as a subrogation analyst, which he explained meant that he investigated health insurance claims; Carter would reach out to patients to learn more about their claims and report back to their insurance company about coverage.

Much like Ava's discussion of how her CNA certification was helping her to contextualize patient experience, Carter's experience as a subrogation analyst led him to a situated perspective on each patient. He explained:

> You know there's always the first initial point of you're dealing with someone's life, their privacy, things of that nature. So, an individual might not know a lot of what's going on with themselves. Or they're going through

testing, and you might see something else [in the test], that's no place for you to go in and step in and just blurt out and tell the individual what's going on. [. . .] You have to look at every individual situation differently. You have to address them differently and [. . .] you still have to learn how to communicate with people.

The points Carter highlights in this initial response were running themes throughout our conversation. He was very hesitant to make broad generalizations about patients, pushing back, for example, when I asked him how he would "prioritize" his patients as a tele-observer. He also was aware of the degree to which he should or should not intervene and what his "place" was in patient interactions. Here, that limit is visible in his discussion of not going in and sharing information from testing with a patient—"step in and just blurt out"—but instead recognizing that his communication with patients will directly affect their emotional and physical state. This is a patient-centered perspective that also relies heavily on Carter's intuitive knowledge of where a patient is at and what they need, his patient sense.

Carter also drew some parallels between his call center work and the technological navigation of the VICU. Juggling multiple people at once on several screens was familiar to him: "Call center wise, you're still dealing with a headset, still have a computer and a keyboard in front of you and a mouse. Just sometimes with the call center you're dealing with about four or five screens instead of just two." And just as the call center work taught him to navigate multiple people on multiple devices, it also reinforced maintaining a degree of distance from the people he was working with. He recognized his own limitations in impacting the mood of the patients, suggesting that emotional modulation was not always possible: "I would say you can't make everybody happy, but you can do your job, do what you're supposed to do, and if they still are not happy or still are not seeing eye to eye, maybe it's not you. Maybe it's something that happened before." Here, again, he is aware of the patient's larger context and experiences as those factors shape their in-the-moment interaction.

Carter's experience with a diverse range of individuals in sales and corporate contexts meant that he was able to distance himself from negative emotional feedback, drawing clear boundaries around what constituted "his job." Overall, while his professional experiences were the most disparate from telework in the group, it was clear that he saw connections in how he managed individuals across contexts as well as the limits of his role when it came to managing their emotions, something not everyone in the group was as strong at recognizing.

Healthcare Experience

As I mentioned, all my interview participants aside from Carter came to the tele-observation role with prior healthcare experience—ranging from working as nursing assistants in hospitals to in-home care to nursing. When I asked about how those prior experiences impacted their work in the VICU, the most direct connection that participants made was how it shaped their understanding of patient experience, and specifically physical patient experience. In fact, Ginny asserted that she believed everyone working in the VICU should spend time on the hospital floor: "It's very easy to get into this position where you're looking at a screen and you're not really feeling like you're there. Because it does seem like you're watching a program or whatever. And I think it's really important to have that awareness of what it's like to be in that room." For interviewees, "that awareness" of the physical experience of the room helped them be more cognizant of what to look out for, as well as how to effectively intervene, supporting them in considering the physical and emotional impact of choices like hitting the stat alarm.

Several participants provided me with specific examples of the ways their physical experiences with patients in healthcare contexts help them to intervene. Becca's experience as a medical aid gave her interventions in the VICU urgency: "If the patient's sitting in the poop, [you] understand, not what the feeling is, but what you should do in a better way. [. . .] I can be quick when I need to." Here, she clarifies that she does not know "what the feeling is" of sitting in feces, but having worked with many patients in that situation, she can also understand that physical experience differently. It is precisely her prior embodied encounters with patients, her physical memory of their discomfort and urgency, that cue her to prioritize fast intervention.

Darilyn described a similar situation during her work in the VICU where one of the patients in her feed had what appeared to be yellow cream on the protective mitts on their hands. She reached out to the nurse on the hospital floor and described the fluid, which was covering the patient's back, shoulders, and mitts. Ultimately, Darilyn's instincts were correct, and the liquid was blood. Reflecting on this experience, Darilyn noted how her experience as a CNA had helped her to sense that something was off, even though the screen distorted the color and texture of the blood.

Frances, whose background included many years working as a nurse, described it succinctly, saying, "It's helpful being a nurse to be able to watch these patients with a better eye." In her example, that better eye included calling a floor nurse when she noticed one of her patients getting red in the face suddenly. She describes her thought process watching this unfold: "Was there a reaction to a medication? Was she getting sick again?" Noticing these "little subtleties" and knowing when they are worth pursuing was key to having a better eye, which was a metaphor Frances used to describe what I would call her intuitive patient sense.

In a similar way, physical exposure to patients that shared the background of those on the screen helped tele-observers be attuned to important physical cues. Evie, who had provided in-home care for patients with traumatic brain injuries, said that she was well aware of how quickly those patients' moods could shift. Watching a patient begin to escalate into agitation on her screen, she described calling in to the nurse who had just entered the room and reflected: "He's started to get more agitated and upset right now and I know many times dealing with that with the resident in their home, I see the same thing happen." Thus, just as formal education and customer service work helped participants contextualize patients with specific backgrounds and conditions, previous healthcare experience also provided this supplemental understanding of the physical experiences of certain kinds of patients. For Evie, understanding how someone with a frontal lobe injury might shift between emotional states was key to her patient sense of the person on the screen and prompted her to follow up with nursing staff effectively.

However, Evie struggled, at times, with convincing nurses of the urgency of her patient's emotional state. She told one story where she was warning a floor nurse that the patient was agitated but the nurse brushed it off. Then, "as she was walking out of the patient's room, he had grabbed a pen off of his bedside table and started to come at her as her back was towards him." This was a terrifying moment for Evie, watching the nurse's safety put at risk as a direct result of failing to attend to the tele-observers' patient sense.

While I discuss the participants' relationships to nurses on the floor in more depth in the next section, this was an area where prior healthcare experience also tended to aid in communication. Ginny was clear that her experience with communication on the hospital floor shaped her interactions with nurses: "I have an advantage that I had worked in the unit with patients and nurses and understand what that communication is." Evie also described how her previous work in home health had prepared her for conversations with nursing staff, as she was accustomed to regular check-ins: "We have to check in with the nurses for those patients that we're monitoring each night, so there's a lot of communication and making sure that we're meeting their needs and their wants with the patient." Knowing how to be in conversation with nurses about patient care, then, was one of her bigger takeaways from previous work. And given her prior experience, she was sympathetic to the heavy patient load nurses carried and the many demands on their time: "you know that they're in a busy setting and that they're taking care of a good amount of patients."

Some of my participants struggled with the physical distance from patients that they experienced in tele-ops. This was the biggest area where their current job diverged from previous work, and it could lead to frustration with physical limitations of the screen. Becca explained that working part-time as a medical assistant and part-time in tele-ops was a good balance for her precisely because of this frustration: "I just like the variety because I'm able to be hands on [as a medical assistant] and be with that person and help them more than trying to just push a staff button or telling the client 'please do not get up' or 'wait for help.'"

For others, the limits on how much they could intervene were a relief, making the job less stressful and less physically exhausting. Frances, who shared that she was sixty-two, noted that her impact on patients was less than it had been as a nurse in the hospital, but the physical toll on her body was also far less: "I was younger and you often did make a difference but [working in the VICU], I'm still helping people, I'm still part of the care team, and I don't have to lift anybody." But for others, it was hard to leave behind the immediate patient access they had had on the hospital floor and accept the physical limits around their current position.

In a similar way, tele-ops had much more restricted access to patient information; they were not able to view the patient chart, likely because of privacy concerns surrounding patient data. Thus, for those who were accustomed to chart access, they often found themselves following up with nurses in the VICU for supplemental information, as well as listening in on patient conversations with the nurse through their headphones. Becca explained:

> You want the background to try to help the person. I don't want to try to be nosy either but sometimes it's just good to know the background because sometimes we have to watch for suspicious behavior of family. So, what are we watching for? Who are we watching for? [...] So that's really hard, trying to pinpoint things, making sure [the patient is] not stabbed and if someone's going to harm the patient making sure [the visitor is] not that person.

This was another area that impacted communication with nurses, as those who had frequent chart access in past jobs better understood the kinds of questions they could ask both nursing staff in the VICU, who could go into patient charts if needed, and nurses on the floor.

I began this section with Carter's comment about drawing on prior work and personal experiences and "incorporate[ing] it all" in his work in the VICU.

As my analysis shows, what it means to incorporate it all—"work, personal, everything in between"—is a complex and multifaceted composite of embodied practices. When tele-observers see a cue from one of their patients that prompts action, they can be drawing on discursive knowledge gained in the classroom about a medical condition, physical knowledge gained in interaction with similar patients on the hospital floor, or even emotional knowledge acquired in customer service interactions. Their patient sense emerges as a composite of these prior experiences, alongside their knowledge and understanding of the VICU's technology. Meanwhile, they develop unique practices of body work that are tailored to this virtual environment. In the next two sections, I consider that rhetorical body work and, specifically, my participants' strategies for patient and interprofessional engagement in the VICU. This section sets the groundwork for recognizing that all those strategies were not created in a vacuum in the VICU but instead are deeply tied to their prior embodied experiences.

Relationships with Patients

When interviewees and I began to discuss their methods for managing patients during day-to-day tele-observation, I was surprised that their range of approaches was as diverse as their ages and professional backgrounds. While nurses will observe and then practice a specific hand maneuver to maintain sterility during a Foley catheter procedure again and again, and PT students will learn how to stimulate a particular muscle to make the hand flex, tele-observers receive ad hoc training and draw primarily on their prior experiences. Thus, their rhetorical body work for patient management was their own—developed out of personal preference in combination with previous knowledge and an awareness of individual positionality. In this section I consider strategies for organizing patients, communicating into the patient's room, and monitoring behavior. I also discuss the wide variety of answers I received to the question "Do you ever wish you could reach through the screen?," which serves as an interesting indicator for how removed or present tele-observers felt with their patients.

Organizing Patients on the Screen

During their shift, tele-observers are typically responsible for tracking six to eight patients, often with a range of conditions. During interviews, I asked how they would organize the different video streams on their screen. There was variety in participant responses with a clear split between those who "prioritized" certain patients (Carter objected to my use of this word, saying that "everybody is prioritized") and those who liked to organize patients in numerical order across the screen. Ava noted, "I just put the most active ones on the top of my screen," and Darilyn agreed, "I would put my really busy patients, I'll put those together." Becca also liked to organize by activity level. Meanwhile, Carter used the numbers on the patient cameras: "Numerical order. Each camera has a number, so I go by the number." Evie and Frances preferred numerical order as well. I did not find out from Ginny her organizational strategy.

Once patient video feeds were organized on the screen, tele-observers would click in and out of patients' rooms to enlarge the video stream and listen in. This was where organizing by activity level could be useful, since tele-ops could spend more time listening to the patients that were visibly active or had providers or family members in the room with them. As Ava explained, "If they're doing nothing then I'll just listen to cameras that are off completely. But if they're active and the nurses are in there then I'll listen." Meanwhile, tele-ops also had a stack of papers to document activity in front of them. Most would match their documentation to their screen organization. Darilyn elaborated, "I will put the patients, the ones that are just irritable, whatever, I will put those papers at the top too, because I know I'm going to need to be marking on those papers more so than others."

In the discrepancies in patient organization, tele-ops' differing values and embodied strategies become apparent. Some of this is likely born from previous professional knowledge and experience, while other choices might emerge as idiosyncratic preferences in response to their physical experience of the VICU. In both cases, however, tele-ops' body work is their own, emergent and responsive to their unique environment.

Documenting Patient Care

Tele-observers' writing on the job consisted of two main tasks using the paper chart that they had for each patient. The first task was to track patient actions hour by hour using a number system that was provided in a box at the bottom of the chart. As Evie explained, "So a number one means they're in the bed. A number three means they're ambulating [walking]. And number four means they're in the bathroom. So, if you see a one, three and a four then you know the patient was in bed and then walked to the bathroom." While clearly open to interpretation, this coding of patient actions seemed transparent on the surface. Evie also explained that over time, the VICU team had added codes to include more specific descriptors: "that list has been changed over the years since I've been there. We didn't always have crying or agitated. We've added to the list just to be a little bit more descriptive." While I did not get more details about the process by which the list was modified or the role that tele-observer feedback played in these revisions, this did point to one way in which the tele-observers had agency to change their writing rules based on their experiential knowledge.

While the numbers system in the tele-observers' charting masqueraded as neutral and objective, it was actually quite flexible and open to interpretation. Evie described a second box for each hour that would elaborate on the patient's mood: "The second box is their mood or what they were doing. Their activity. So, for that you would put calm, sleeping, active, restless, impulsive. Restless is another one, that's different than impulsive." At this point in the interview, I stopped Evie so that we could dig into the language she was using. "Impulsive" seemed like an outlier on the list she was giving, both because it had more negative than neutral connotations and because it seemed more tied to personality than to actions. Evie explained that the notes section on their chart would help them to unpack the impulsive code: "So that's the thing, if you would put impulsive down then that's when it's different in the note section. 'Patient very active under his covers' or 'Patient reaching up on the back wall at cords.' That's when it's sometimes good to put what they were doing." Therefore, the notes section of the chart gave tele-observers a chance to personalize their coding system and in some cases to even justify their coding choices. The notes also served a definitional function, in explaining a coding choice, the tele-observers were also creating and reinforcing its meaning.

Despite the clearly meticulous writing work that the tele-ops put into charting patient actions, I never received a clear answer on what happened to all their paper charting. The charts were certainly used during hand-offs to help update an incoming tele-observer about the status of each patient. They also played an important role in justifying the removal of a camera from a patient on the floor, as I discuss below. Ava assured me that "we hand [the charting] off to someone else who will then upload it to [the patients'] records," but without much clarity on who that person was or how this activity fit into the larger workflow of the VICU. Thus, tele-observers' documentation is part of a larger system of devaluing their work and expertise. In her article "Who Has the Right to Write?," Marotta argues that institutions, in her case the university, strategically conscript who has the access and ability to produce writing to reinforce racial and professional hierarchies. Meanwhile, by isolating tele-observers' writing from the electronic patient health records used by other providers, tele-observers' professional knowledge and patient sense is not recorded in hospital systems, contributing to its devaluing.

Patient Communication

Once patients and their paperwork were organized, tele-ops also had strategies for intervening to redirect patient behavior. Here, I found quite a bit of variation in how often the observers would rely on a stat alarm, use their own voice in the room, or use an automatic recorded voice. In general, the group agreed on a protocol of escalation that began with a verbal or automated redirect, progressed to calling the nurse on duty, and then escalated to using the stat alarm so that the closest provider would come and assist the patient.

Several tele-observers described using the patient's name in an initial redirect, modeling language for me. Evie described a possible patient response: "Richard, you have to stop touching that. Please don't touch that." Similarly, Frances demonstrated a patient conversation, saying, "Okay, Jane. Please put your legs back in the bed. What can I help you with? I can get someone to help you." Ava explained that by using patients' names it was clear that the tele-observers' instructions were directed at them. This was particularly important for disoriented patients: "sometimes they're confused on who you're talking to or sometimes they don't realize the camera's there, so you're just trying to get their attention."

Other tele-ops preferred using automated redirects, however, rather than using their own voice to speak to the patient. Darilyn, for example, said she relied heavily on the automated voice for instructions like "Do not touch that" or "Don't get out of bed." Darilyn would only use her own voice if there was not an appropriate automated message available, because in her view patients responded better to the audio recording. Meanwhile, Evie said she would use the automated voice as a second resort, if the patient seemed unclear on her verbal directions or unwilling to comply: "Other times patients will be like, 'What? I didn't hear you. What did you say?' so then I'll just use the automated voice where it says [deepens her voice], 'Attention please stop what you are doing.' But then it's a robot and sometimes then they're like, 'Oh, okay, alright.' And then they'll stop what they're doing. Sometimes it takes that robot voice." It was interesting to me that both women associated the robotic voice with an additional degree of authority, so that even though it depersonalized the patient interaction, it could also lead to greater compliance. The disadvantage was that it could be unclear to a patient that the directive was for them at all and could be disorienting to an already confused patient.

Ginny expressed similar concerns about using the stat alarm, which she said she tried to use minimally because of its potential to upset patients. She noted that she was told to use the stat alarm regularly during training—"it was almost like do that more than thinking about anything else"—but she has come to question its usefulness, wondering if the negative effects outweighed the positive. She mentioned that she has brought up to their boss the risk of overrelying on the alarm, when "you may be creating more of a situation where the patient is more agitated." In general, Ginny wanted to respond contextually to different patients' needs, a desire that was shared by many of the other observers, especially Carter and Frances.

Ginny explained that for a "little old lady [. . .] who is confused about why they're there in the first place," they are often happy to have someone to talk to and answer questions, but for a schizophrenic or someone with trust issues, the experience of a voice coming from the ceiling is deeply upsetting. She noted that for some patients, nurses and tele-ops have come to an understanding that it is better not to talk to them at all. Here, the discursive body work of the tele-op is modified both in response to their own positionality (i.e., do patients respond well when they issue directives?) and to the patient's emotional and physical state. Understanding when and where to leverage the different verbal modes available to them depends in large part on the tele-op's patient sense and especially their reliance on embodied patient cues.

Embodied Patient Cues

In line with this focus on contextual care, tele-ops also described for me what they are watching for in patient behavior to cue their interventions. Several of them noted that their observations are tied to notes about individual patient diagnoses. As Becca explained: "So 'fall risk,' if the patient's trying to get up. If they're trying to take off their mitts or restraints, things for holding them down, take the side rail off. Or if we're watching for safety of tubes and lines, if they're picking, scratching, under the covers moving. If they're for suicide, just any forms of tools in their room." Since they could be watching six to eight patients with different diagnoses, tele-ops would have to rapidly switch between individualized patient concerns as they moved from video stream to video stream.

At the same time, a few tele-ops noted that patients would occasionally lull them into a false sense of security, seeming calm and placated for hours and then quickly becoming active. Frances described a patient who went from sleeping to bolting from his bed in a matter of seconds. As soon as he sat up, she had to be attuned and ready to respond: "I mean it's so quick [...] the minute he sits up I'm like 'okay,' but if you miss that suddenly he's bolting across the room, right?" Similarly, Ginny described a patient who had been engaging in a repeated ritual of behaviors, moving around the room consistently for six hours. Then, he suddenly unplugged the camera and was out the door. She reflected, "I actually saw that happen and I thought, 'that person was aware of me for six hours and probably planning this the whole time.'"

Because shifts in behavior can be so sudden, tele-ops must be exceptionally attentive to minor changes in emotional or physical comportment, cued into any slight shift that might indicate the patient is about to escalate behavior. In Ginny's view, much of this attunement happens at preconscious levels, as is often true of patient sense. This makes it difficult to articulate exactly what she is watching for: "I think as human beings we communicate on so many levels that we're not even aware of. So it could just be the facial expression on someone that you've been watching that, because you've been watching them for eight hours, you notice a change and then you'll click on that room." This patient sense also requires experience and training to recognize, so that newer tele-ops might struggle to figure out what they missed when a patient suddenly changes course.

Reaching through the Screen

One of the last questions that I asked tele-ops during our interviews was whether there was ever a moment when they wanted to "reach through the screen" to intervene with one of the patients they were observing. Much like the question about patient organization, responses were split nearly fifty-fifty among my participants. Ava, Carter, and Darilyn all said "no" while Becca, Evie, Frances, and Ginny all said "yes." Folks in the "no" camp emphasized the need to keep boundaries between themselves and the patients, especially because they were not capable of physically intervening. For example, Ava noted that her instinct when a patient needed intervention was to try to get a nurse there quickly. However, she emphasized, "I try not to take this home with me because we're not doing so much for them emotionally." Like many of my participants, Ava also worked as a CNA in a nursing home, where it was more challenging to draw clear emotional boundaries with patients.

Meanwhile, Darilyn expressed some sadness about her futility, "You just wish that they wouldn't do things, you know certain things, hurt themselves.

I just act as urgently as I can to help them." One trend among my "no" group was that they had not been working in the VICU as long on average. Ava and Carter had been there about a year, while Darilyn had only been there two months. This is too small a group to draw broader conclusions from, but I was interested that in my interviews, extended time in the VICU did not seem to reinforce distancing from patients like one might expect. This could also be an observation about the type of person who was likely to continue working in the VICU long-term, someone who was emotionally invested in the patients on the screen.

Among my "yes" participants, several observers noted their frustration with the speed of response on the hospital floor. They wanted to reach through the screen so that they could intervene more quickly and more effectively than the providers they were alerting. In her response, Becca repeated twice that she "want[ed] to help more": "If they're going to fall, I want to kind of catch them, but the stat alarm doesn't really work because most times in two of the hospitals they can't run there fast enough." Evie similarly noted that sometimes when she has called an alarm on a patient, it felt like she was watching the response in slow motion: "They're not getting in there fast enough and it's like, 'Come on, get in there!!' You're jumping out of your seat like 'Hurry!' like you're watching it on some movie." The comparison to a movie is a notable one, especially because Evie was someone who ultimately expressed a lot of connection and concern for her patients. However, at crucial moments, she cannot break the barrier of the screen and is left yelling on the sidelines, hoping the hospital team will come through. Clearly, despite the physical distance, her emotional investment and response is very high. Because she is not physically present with the patient or family members, she also does not have to modulate this emotional response to the same degree either.

There was a sense among the "yes" group that they did have a lot of investment in patient well-being, perhaps more than would be ideal in some cases. Frances, who had worked for years as a nurse, lamented that she could not be more physically present with patients in need or when a friend or family member was behaving badly: "I just want to say, 'Okay I'll just wait here with you until somebody comes.'" Meanwhile, Ginny acknowledged that she struggled to leave the emotional baggage of her job at work. Early on in her time in the VICU, she could not help but think about patients: "I went home and thought about them and worried that I wasn't going to be able to do this job." This was not new for Ginny, however, who explained that early in her career when she considered becoming a nurse, a head nurse had told her, "You're not going to make a good nurse if you don't know how to detach." Ginny said it took most of her career to understand what that meant. The VICU presented an ideal workplace for her because she did not have direct contact with patients and there was some emotional distance, but she was still able to help and provide support, even if she did struggle to leave work at work.

Relationship-building with patients looks different when mediated through a video screen and a microphone. And yet, the presence of rhetorical body work was no less visible for tele-ops than it might be on a hospital floor. Tele-observers made strategic embodied choices in their use of voice and tone and their engagement with automated voices and alarms. They carefully read their patients' physical cues, relying on patient sense to inform their decision-making about interventions. And for some, they felt deeply emotionally connected to their patients, physically responding, and even yelling on the sidelines while they waited for hospital nurses to intervene. I am reminded of Maura's experiences during simulations, where she too became physically and emotionally connected to the experiences of the patient manikin despite her lack of physical presence in the room with students. Both examples demonstrate the way that providers experience mediated technological patient connections in their bodies, engaging in a transformed form of body work, but one that is no less affecting or motivating.

Interprofessional Engagement

In addition to interactions with patients, cooperating with the nursing team on the hospital floor required tele-observers to engage in a range of rhetorical body work as well. They modulated their emotions, tone, and word choice to establish a collaborative relationship; relied on their patient sense as primary evidence; and accessed additional information through collaboration with nurses in the VICU as well as careful observation and "listening in" on their patients. In this section, I overview four points of conflict between the floor nurses and tele-observers—access to patient information, camera placement, trusting tele-ops' patient sense, and missed cues—and then draw on my interviews to discuss how tele-observers navigated these conflicts using their range of embodied knowledge.

Access to Patient Information

Because tele-observers were not able to access patients' charts, their incoming patient knowledge came primarily from the previous tele-observer, who would hand off their patients and documentation at the end of their shift, and from the nursing team on the hospital floor. However, nurses on the floor were on a twelve-hour shift and tele-ops were on an eight-hour shift, so their hand-offs did not easily align. Typically, tele-observers would check in with the nurses responsible for their patients about forty-five minutes to an hour into the tele-observation shift. At that point, nurses were occasionally frustrated at the disruption or disinterested in exchanging information. Evie explained: "[Nurses] will be like, 'I already read this' or 'I heard this earlier,' you know? But we have to read that script each shift. So that can be hard sometimes because they're like, 'Oh, here we go.' And then many times they'll even talk in the background to somebody else. It's like that's rude, but whatever." Information access creates a disconnect; while the tele-ops rely on floor nurses to provide them with patient insights they cannot access in a chart, the floor nurses do not have a similar knowledge gap that they need filled by the tele-ops. This makes the exchange feel unnecessary on their end, leading to some frustration as both groups navigate a mandated conversation.

On the other hand, tele-observers described having to frequently check in with nurses to get updates because it was unusual that a nurse would reach out to them to let them know about an intervention or change in patient care. Evie explained, "they rarely ever call us to tell us that they put something new in" and noted how this could affect not only her but also the person she handed off care to. For example, if the nurse puts in a Foley without contacting the team and it is not noted in a patient's record, then Evie described that "the next shift coming on doesn't know that the patient has a Foley and if he's messing around under the covers they're thinking 'the patient doesn't have anything under there.'" Therefore, the tele-observers could not count on nurses to be keeping them up to date on the patient's status, and without access to the patient's chart, they relied instead on other kinds of relational strategies to get patient information. This included building trusting relationships with the nursing team both on the floor and in the VICU, as well as listening in on patient conversations with providers on the floor for additional context.

As with other professions overviewed in this book, power differentials were noticeable in the VICU setting. Interactions with nurses on the floor were governed by a power imbalance, in terms of educational training and prestige, which I discuss below, but also in terms of information access. Tele-observers had to balance the instinct to not bother very busy floor nurses with their need for information and patient updates. Several of them described how developing a trusting relationship with nurses was key to making this dynamic successful, as well as always asking for additional insights beyond the basics during the hand-off. For example, Ginny noted how her last question in the hand-off was always "'Is there anything else that you find that you're concerned about?' and just asking that question I've found that the nurses are much more apt to call if there's something that they've noticed or maybe bring up something they wouldn't have just normally brought up." Ginny's phrasing focuses on the nurse's experience, "you," rather than herself (i.e., "Is there anything else I should know?"), a savvy rhetorical move to elevate the nurse's perspective and concerns. Similarly, when tele-ops saw nurses providing care that might include something like a new tube or line, they would often reach out directly to ask what changes had been made.

In addition to encouraging the floor nurses to share extra insights with them, tele-ops would also occasionally ask nurses in the VICU for information from a patient's chart or listen into conversations in the room. As Frances explained, "we're given this very basic information but oftentimes you can hear it from conversations or whatever what may have happened or is happening." When they shared this with me, several of the tele-ops were apologetic, emphasizing that they were not trying to be nosy or violate the patient's privacy. It was just that learning, for example, that there was a conflict with a family member through a conversation between nurse and patient could be vital information to help tele-ops know that they should be on high alert when family members were in the room. Carter elaborated, "You have to kind of listen in on those particular type of things. Not to use it against them but just to know what type of situation you're dealing with." Overall, I found that the tele-ops relied heavily on emotional modulation with floor nurses and on listening to patient conversations to supplement their limited information access.

Camera Placement

Another source of conflict between tele-ops and nurses on the floor was which patients should receive or keep a camera in their room. For high-risk patients, some nurses preferred having an extra pair of eyes to support their care continuously. However, the tele-ops had specific protocols for how long to keep a camera in a patient's room. Ava explained that the tele-ops have a behavior list, and when a patient has been on good behavior for twenty-four hours, then the camera should be removed. However, because nurses are only interacting with patients over a twelve-hour shift, they may not be familiar with that history of good behavior and will sometimes argue to keep the camera. Other times, they might say that a patient is on suicide watch when that is not in the tele-op's record. As Bella noted, "'Are they really suicide or do [the nurses] just really want the camera?' So, we just have to watch the patient until the [VICU] nurses check that out." This puts tele-ops in the position of having to inform nurses that the camera must be removed, a difficult conversation given the power dynamics between the groups.

Becca explained that tele-ops can use a script to notify nurses that a camera is being removed. This script uses directive language to describe the removal rather than a question, circumventing any confusion and helping to counter power differentials between the groups: "'Your patient has had very little interventions in the last 24 hours so we're going to pull the camera.' And most times they'll say, 'Well, we have a doctor's order' or 'We had interventions' but they're not on our sheet, so we just have our [VICU] nurses take a look at that and we'll give them a call back." In Becca's explanation, the role of the VICU nurses in camera removal is also visible. Since tele-ops only have records of interventions that the nurses have updated them on, they may have gaps in their knowledge. Therefore, the VICU nurses must check a patient's chart to confirm that there have not been interventions in the last twenty-four hours. Ava also described bringing older tele-ops into the conversation when a nurse argued about camera removal, especially when she was new to the position. In both cases, the tele-ops gain legitimacy by leveraging their relationships with others in the VICU to support them during a difficult conversation with nurses on the floor.

Trusting the Tele-Ops

Something nursing instructors discussed often when I was observing clinical simulations was how much more patient knowledge nurses had than other providers because they are frequently in contact with the patient—physically in the room with them, palpating them, asking them questions, getting to know them as individuals. Thus, I was surprised that some nurses did not recognize that tele-ops have a similar degree of patient knowledge because they are present with the patient constantly throughout the day. The virtual element of tele-monitoring might contribute to its devaluing, with nurses questioning whether tele-ops could really know a patient through a screen. However, educational differences were also clearly at play, as was informational access, in some of the mistrust that nurses had for tele-ops' perspectives.

Evie captures the differing levels of access and expertise that informed decision-making and communication between tele-ops and nurses: "[The nurse] is just seeing that patient for a few minutes at a time, dropping into the patient's room to hand them something or help them with something and then she's back out, where I'm monitoring that patient that whole time. So, I'm the one who has, I guess not more education, not a better/higher degree, but I'm witnessing and noticing more." Tele-ops struggled with this combination. Most of them did not have the educational background of nurses nor access to a chart that would give them information about a patient's diagnosis. And yet, they often knew these patients very intimately from near-constant surveillance and were therefore attuned to minor changes in physical or emotional states. Therefore, when they would call a nurse to alert them about a problematic change in patient behavior, they had to rely on claims of intuition or embodied knowledge that are often not as persuasive in medical contexts that favor data-driven arguments (Campbell and Angeli). This, combined with the fact that many of the nurses prided themselves on having a thick skin and were, as Evie described it, "not as afraid as they should be at times," meant that the tele-ops could find themselves in the position of having their concerns about a patient dismissed. Evie's story about the patient who nearly stabbed the nurse with a pen even after Evie gave a warning that he seemed agitated is a prime example of this dismissal. Others had less dire stories, but still described times when they had to argue firmly—and sometimes with intervention from a VICU nurse—to get floor nurses to take their concerns about patient safety seriously.

Recognizing the power dynamics at play, most of the tele-ops that I talked to said that the answer to these conflicts was primarily respect and an acknowledgment of the many challenges that floor nurses were facing. Tele-ops with hospital experience had a good deal of empathy for nurses juggling many patients and knew what it was like to question reports coming from someone in a virtual role. At the same time, tele-ops did not shy away from reporting concerns, even if they knew they might face resistance. Ginny mentioned receiving advice from their boss during training: "Any time you feel something doesn't feel right, don't question it! Just call the nurse. Just do that extra thing." She said that she thinks of this often because it is easy to question herself and her insights.

Ginny also described how tele-ops lean on one another to support their intuition about patient safety and build the confidence to report problems: "And I've heard this with my co-workers too. [. . .] They'll say 'That person's breathing is so different,' 'Look at the color in their face,' and they'll say, 'Would you mind clicking the camera and tell me what you think? Is this unusual?' and [. . .] so many times they've been right on." These small changes that the tele-ops are attuned to, Ginny asserts, show up before the data-oriented tracking on the floor—before the telemetry machines know that a patient is crashing, for example, or the nurse's station will receive an alert.

In those moments, the tele-ops' virtual patient knowledge still constitutes patient sense, attuned to individual differences between patients and more alert to small shifts and changes in bodies and in emotional states than even the best equipment. At the same time, making sure that this patient sense is recognized and valued by their professional collaborators requires a good deal of emotional body work to navigate challenging conversations across power imbalances.

Missed Signals

While it was clear to me from conversations with the tele-ops that they offered valuable insights into patients' well-being, it was also undeniable that it was challenging for them to keep track of six to eight high-risk patients at all times. As Becca explained, with this many patients to watch "you always miss something." Conflicts tended to arise from these missed signals because the nurses did not always understand tele-ops' patient load and were occasionally under the impression that they, like the sitters that preceded them, were watching a single patient. Ginny explained:

> Because I've had nurses call and say, "You didn't see that happening?!" and I said, "You know I could have been dealing with a very difficult patient that was almost falling out of the bed." And I'll say to them, [. . .] "Honestly, at the moment that that was happening in your room, I was dealing with another situation and I'm sorry, but I didn't catch it." And they—in most cases they'll understand that.

The strategy for tele-ops then, was to help contextualize their jobs for the nurses on the floor. Since many of them had hospital floor experience, it was easy for them to imagine why the nurses were harried or pulled in many directions. They also recognized that their own roles might be perceived as cushy or relaxed in comparison. Ginny emphasized this need for mutual respect and understanding between providers: "I think on both sides, the tele-operator can have an assumption about what's going on on that floor and the nurses on the floor can have assumptions that we've got this real easy job that we're just sitting back and watching people, having a great time, not really watching the patients." Therefore, tele-ops had to educate the nursing team on their role and the various responsibilities they held while also maintaining respect for the challenges of the nurse's role.

For the most part, tele-ops reported that providing context to the nurses about where their attention might be pulled when they missed something with a patient was sufficient. However, sometimes this would not satisfy a nurse and she would report the miss to the tele-ops' supervisor. In these cases, the tele-ops' handwritten records of patient events became a primary source of evidence. As Ginny explained, "if we've written down an adverse event report and then told our manager and 'yeah this happened, this is just like a slip here but unavoidable, an unavoidable slip,' then that is enough explanation."

Overall, the tele-ops relied on positive will from the nurses when errors were made. They worked hard to contextualize their own work environment, recognize the many challenges facing the floor nurses, and create a relationship built on mutual trust and respect. However, they were often working against a general mistrust born of educational difference, difference in physical proximity, and occasionally assumptions about working-class employees that informed nurses' responses (Rose). Ginny, who had worked on the floor in an EEG room, reported that the talk about tele-observers among nurses often skewed negative: "When I was in EEG and I heard about tele-monitoring and we had these cameras on the floor, they were complaining, 'Oh well they missed that' or 'Oh that camera is constantly going off.' You get this impression that people are really not into their job, because they're missing things." Tele-ops struggled to counter these assumptions and stand up for the validity of their insights even if errors were made.

While there are many barriers to successful communication between nurses and tele-ops, I want to end on a positive note, considering what it looks like when the two kinds of providers can draw on their differing but complementary patient sense to optimize patient care. Ginny told a story of a patient who was always pulling on her tracheal tube and at one point had a male visitor. Initially, Ginny thought the visitor was helping the patient take off her mitts, something that is often allowed. However, the visitor was standing in front of the camera and when he moved, Ginny realized that the patient's tracheal tube had been removed. She reported this to the supervising nurse, who asked detailed questions about the patient's physical strength and ability to remove the trach herself. At the end of the conversation, Ginny said it was clear that "something had clicked" for the nurse in terms of understanding, and while she did not know about the outcome, Ginny was satisfied with how the conversation had gone: "If she's liable for something going on, she wants to know what steps led up to it."

In this instance, the nurse's willingness to engage with the tele-op's patient sense—acquired from multiple days of constant surveillance and intuitive attention to the patient—provided her new insight into the patient's state. This allowed the nurse to better protect the patient going forward and to have more contextualized knowledge of the patient's condition than she could get from the chart or machine monitoring. The tele-ops' body work, then, includes not just the physical and emotional knowledge that they acquire and hold regarding the patients they observe, but also emotional modulation used to preserve their relationships with nurses on the hospital floor so that their patient sense will be taken seriously going forward.

Physical Experience of the Job

Most of my participants described their work in the VICU as calm, not emotional, and not physically demanding. Compared with previous jobs they had working on the hospital floor—as receptionists, CNAs, and even nurses—the pace of the VICU was slow. Only Ginny mentioned physical symptoms that emerged from the stress of the job, noting that in her first month of work, "I started having stomach issues, because it was so real." She attributed this stress reaction both to the severity of her patients' conditions—having multiple patients on suicide watch, for example—and to her inability to distance herself from the job at the end of the day.

Ginny found that turning to her co-workers for support was key to adapting to the position and coping with the stress. When administrators from the overseeing hospital came to talk to the tele-ops about their jobs because they wanted to integrate a tele-op position into a mental health wing, Ginny was adamant that they should hire more than one person, telling them: "I think that it's very important that somebody has another person with them when they're doing this." Other participants agreed that their amicable relationship with one another in the VICU was a key contributor to their quality of life. While a few found the level of background noise in the VICU room somewhat stressful, they were glad to have co-workers and nurses nearby to check in with and trade off patient observation to take breaks.

Physically, the main drawback of the job is its sedentary nature, especially for observers who might be used to much more movement in the workplace. On a long shift or working in the evening, eating and drinking were popular strategies for staying awake. Darilyn commented, "I can always have something to drink. I'm trying not to eat too much." Carter agreed that the main downside of the job was just the availability of snacks, especially when they were spending so much time sitting: "Lot of sweets. Eating a lot of sweets. All this time to find stuff to munch on and you can't munch and sit." Similarly, Evie, who had been working there for five years, noted: "I have gained some weight, too much." However, she followed up with: "It's not like somebody is holding us down in our chairs either."

Most of the interviewees commented on the various supports that were offered to them to keep them moving. Desks could be raised for standing; the VICU had weights available and small exercise bikes that could be positioned under the desks. However, I did not observe tele-ops using the exercise equipment, perhaps because they found it challenging to be moving while on the job. Frances, the former nurse who was also an avid traveler and mountain biker, was the exception and said she frequently used the different weights and did squats in the VICU. She noted, "I don't sit down much. [. . .] The nurses stand a lot too. But it's really, yeah because I do a lot of—I do mountain biking and stuff and I really need the upper-body strength." Since Frances only worked about eight days a month and spent the rest of her time biking and traveling, she had a clear motivation to stay in shape and make use of the available equipment.

However, for many of my participants the limited physical activity of the job was a main draw, especially after long careers of active work. Several older participants considered the tele-op job a kind of retirement plan, a job they could continue for the foreseeable future precisely because it did not have significant physical demands and came with health insurance. Frances summarized this attitude, saying: "I'm 62, I could see working there for a very long time unless something stopped me medically. I have part-time hours, I have benefits, I enjoy the job." Ginny, who was also retirement-age and worked part-time hours, agreed that she could see continuing in the VICU for a long time: "I couldn't retire, so this is kind of my pre-retirement plan if I'm going to ever truly retire." Carter and Darilyn, who were middle-aged, expressed a similar view of the future, mentioning that they could see staying in the position long-term. Evie agreed, citing the physical toll that her previous roles in healthcare had taken on her body: "I feel like I did my fair share of like physical work and stuff like that and I don't have the greatest back and hips." Alluding here to a third definition of body work, the physical impact on the worker's body (Gimlin), it's clear that the VICU offers an alternative career path for healthcare professionals who have previously worked jobs that make huge demands on their bodies. By shifting body work into a virtual context, providers can draw on the physical and intuitive knowledge of previous body work, but in a space with fewer physical demands.

On the other hand, many individuals use the VICU job as a stepping stone to other career paths. Becca mentioned that having been a tele-op for four and a half years, she had seen extensive turnover in the department, colleagues moving to different hospitals, graduating, or retiring. In my group of participants, both Ava and Becca were in school. Ava was a traditional college-age student enrolled in a BA program in biology with plans to pursue genetic counseling training, and Becca was in her thirties and pursuing a master's degree in social work. Still, Becca asserted she "would never leave" the VICU, since she had seen how much flexibility the position could offer for retirement-aged workers with a part-time schedule.

I began the chapter with the assertion that the tele-observers' body work cannot be easily replaced by an algorithm or an international worker thousands of miles away. As I have demonstrated, tele-ops' patient sense emerges at an intersection of discursive, classroom-based learning; physical and emotional client interactions in a wide range of previous professional contexts ranging from healthcare to customer service; and experiential knowledge of the technologies in the VICU and their various affordances and limitations. Thus, when a tele-op makes the call to "trust their gut" and notify a floor nurse about a suspicious liquid that is visible on their patient's neck and upper torso, the wide range of expertise and embodied knowledge that informs that decision is nearly impossible to articulate, let alone capture in an algorithm. While we can perhaps imagine automated sensors that could give tele-ops helpful data about patient experiences to supplement this patient sense, like Sauer ("Embodied Knowledge") describes, the future of tele-observation must be one that allows for two-way communication between bodies and machines.

As Ginny was quick to emphasize as well, the future of tele-observation should not be one that features lone tele-observers and their computers. Tele-observers relied on one another as well as the nurses in the VICU to fill in the gaps in their patient knowledge caused by limited chart access, to affirm their embodied expertise and support their decisions, and to provide emotional support and comfort in the wake of difficult patient interactions. Their rhetorical body work was made possible by the collaborative and connected interpersonal environment of the VICU. Thus, this job would not look the same if it featured a single, isolated individual, and while hospitals may be quick to try to cut back employees or outsource this work to reduce expenses, this research points to the necessity of maintaining a social environment for tele-ops. The collaborative environment of the VICU reinforced their patient sense and supported their emotional navigation of interprofessional conversations.

In addition, visible in this discussion is the vital role that prior experiences play in informing the body work of tele-observers. They draw on embodied patient knowledge from previous healthcare experiences but also on emotional knowledge of how to navigate difficult conversations with both superiors and clients. Thus, my analysis has implications for how we approach professionalizing telehealth workers in positions that are outside formal degree programs. My findings reinforce the necessity of on-the-job training and experiences that will put students physically into hospital rooms and other healthcare contexts, which is critical as virtual training and online certifications grow in popularity.

This chapter also points to the need to value perspectives from those whose training has occurred outside of traditional college credentialing in both technical communication research and in certification systems (Campbell, "Not Just Doctors"). Biases in academic research tend to privilege research and perspectives from traditional students and white-collar professionals (Rose). Meanwhile, tele-ops' writing is cordoned off from the rest of the writing activities in the hospital, reserved only for an audience of one another. In line with Marotta's argument, they are not given the "right to write," at least not for those beyond their immediate professional circle. This devaluing of their writing compounds their potential precarity because their knowledge and skills are not documented or encoded into the hospital's day-to-day practices. However, tele-ops' perspectives can expand our field's understanding of both what constitutes professional knowledge and how it is developed and maintained through embodied processes. Or, as Carter put it, these experiences might help us to value and encourage our students to value "anything that keeps the learning going," recognizing how their extracurricular activities (Rifenburg) and service jobs (Brittenham)—among other things—contribute to rhetorical body work that is neither purely discursive nor linear.

CONCLUSION

Body Matters for the Future of Healthcare and Technology

In the opening to *The Doctor and the Algorithm,* Graham offers multiple perspectives on the rise of AI in healthcare—the pessimistic versions that highlight the inherent biases and stereotypes that are embedded in AI systems (Benjamin; Noble) and the more optimistic takes on how AI might serve to humanize medical care. Summarizing Topol's optimistic take, Graham says, "When AI frees physicians from the administrative burdens of electronic medical records, reading lab results, and performing analyses, then they will be better able to provide patients with the emotional labor so often lacking in contemporary medicine" (7). What is interesting to me here and what I take up in this conclusion is the inherent separation between rhetorical labor and emotional labor that this statement sets out. By eliminating the rhetorical labor of doctors (electronic medical records, interpretation of lab results, analyses of data), Topol argues that doctors create space for emotional work.

However, as a rhetorical theory of body work demonstrates, these divisions are not so simple. We cannot expect to offload our rhetorical work onto algorithms or remote workers and still be able to perform the embodied and emotional labor that constitutes rhetorical body work. The documentation in electronic medical records, the interpretation of results: these are physical and emotion-filled tasks, guided by intuition, by prior knowledge, by embodied experience. And empathetic interactions with patients are highly rhetorical tasks, embedded in a deep awareness of audience and context that is tied to the interpretive patient knowledge that practitioners gain from their work. This is perhaps even more visible in the allied health professions, where the body is rarely cordoned off into parts as Wolkowitz describes ("Social Relations" 501) and instead must be both understood and communicated holistically.

Thus, I conclude by returning to my three research questions from the introduction and considering the transformations and constants that emerge at the intersection of rhetorical body work and new health technologies. Overall, I emphasize that rhetorical work *is* body work and body work *is* rhetorical work. By highlighting the inherent interconnections between these concepts, we can begin to speak back to arguments in favor of offloading rhetorical and embodied labor onto machines and algorithms in the future, highlighting the risks of that approach.

Disciplinary Knowledge and Body Work

Each body chapter emphasized a key component of embodied, emotional, and discursive practice that is central to the field's identity. In nursing, I demonstrated how *empathy* takes on a primary role in student learning alongside robotic patient manikins; being able to understand and identify with patient experience is understood as primary to nursing practice. Lessons about empathy manifest in clinical nursing simulations, as instructors design physical, emotional, and discursive cues to prompt students to engage empathetically with their robotic patients. These cues create imperfect lessons in patient sense as the robotic manikin is too large, too stiff, too male, and so forth. However, the simulation's disruptions also help support student responsiveness, prompting reflection and revision of engrained embodied and emotional practices.

In physical therapy, the field's historic relationship to mainstream biomedicine shapes its ongoing quest for legitimacy and professional recognition. Thus, rhetorical body work serves as boundary-work, reifying PTs' professional *expertise* and distinguishing them from complementary and alternative medicine. Efforts to professionalize PTs' patient sense emerge in both explicit lessons on physical interactions with and without technology and in the hidden curriculum of the lab. Overall, PTs are taught that their expertise is crucial to their professional identity, and they learn to enact this expertise through their physical, emotional, and discursive comportment. At times, however, this emphasis on expertise overshadows the field's holistic attention to individual patient experience.

Finally, tele-observers bring to their practice a great deal of intuitive patient knowledge, acquired both in complementary hospital contexts and from other educational and workplace experiences. As they watch patient actions mediated by a video camera and microphone, they learn to "trust their gut" when something seems off about a patient and rely on *intuition* to shape their decisions about intervention. This intuition emerges at an intersection between their prior embodied knowledge and the physical patient actions that are mediated by their screens. It is reinforced in conversation with colleagues, challenged by floor nurses, and at times, must be defended or justified using discursive and emotional rhetorical body work.

All three cases demonstrate how rhetorical body work emerges at an intersection between field-specific knowledge and embodied practices, challenging any assumptions that we can address these two components independently. Empathy, expertise, and intuition are all deeply embodied forms of professional knowledge that rely on experience alongside disciplinary understanding. For rhetorical scholars, I hope these cases demonstrate the value of studying disciplinary learning through an embodied, material framework. While several recent books on professional communication incorporate ethnographic approaches (Angeli; Britt; Fountain; Mackiewicz), there is still ample opportunity for exploration. In rhetoric of health and medicine, I urge scholars to move beyond a focus on doctors, to consider the numerous allied health providers whose rhetorical body work is uniquely tied to their professional discourses, values, and patient sense.

In addition, future educators must consider how they can integrate both providers' and patients' bodies into the teaching of technical knowledge in their disciplines. They must be wary of overemphasizing biomedical knowledge which—while it might help to accrue prestige and recognition professionally—also risks devaluing patient sense. Perhaps this is an unnecessary call for the health sciences, since my research demonstrates that embodied practice is central to experiential learning in fields like nursing and physical therapy. However, as programs move toward online and distance education, it is an important reminder of how imperative physical presence and emotional interaction are to learning in the health sciences. And for tele-observers, their prior in-person professional experiences directly impacted their practice and patient sense. Thus, my findings reinforce the necessity of on-the-job training and experiences that will put students physically into hospital rooms and other healthcare contexts prior to working in virtual spaces.

Technological Mediation of Patient Sense

Often, a primary concern as we move into technological spaces is that these virtual contexts remove the need for critical engagement or reflection. Indeed, we see this anxiety in conversations about large language models like ChatGPT, where teachers bemoan the possibility that students will let the machines do all the difficult thinking involved with writing (Vee). As a writing teacher, I certainly share these concerns about outsourcing the intellectual labor of writing. However, I am also heartened by the fact that all three of my case studies demonstrated the reverse; technological mediation led to a greater need for critical engagement and reflection by destabilizing students' and practitioners' habitual actions.

Lapum et al. articulate this argument in their call for a cyborg ontology for healthcare. They describe both the fears about inattention and complacency that emerge in relationship to technological ways of being, and also the potential for disruption:

> The inherent danger is that a mere technological, habitual way of being does not permit us to be open to the embodied and contextualized experiences of patients. A disruption of the habitual in terms of logics, embodiment, and routines can move nurses and other healthcare professionals to a conscious integration of [person-centered practice] into the technological care environments. (286)

The idea of disruptions as effectively redirecting habitual actions has shown up in both scholarship on Burke and the body (Hawhee, *Moving Bodies*) as well as in simulation scholarship (Magelssen). Phronesis has also been understood as disruptive and a force of resistance against technological complacency (Smith). However, my emphasis on health technology's disruptive potential helps consider new sources of disruption in students' acquisition of rhetorical body work.

In my discussion of nursing simulations, I focus on the manikin as a key source of disruption. Its inability to perfectly replicate a human body or provide students with an exact approximation of patient sense contributed to numerous opportunities for reflection and response. Similarly, I argue that the technologies in the PT lab both promote attention, as students navigate concerns about the technology's physical impact on their partners, and highlight bodily difference, as students learn to recognize different capacities for pain tolerance or mobility in one another. Finally, while tele-observation was my most technologically mediated field site, my interviews with tele-ops demonstrated a complex and responsive rhetorical knowledge that was engaged in every decision they made—from speaking directly to a patient instead of using a recorded voice to calling for nurse intervention when they noticed an unidentified liquid on the patient through the screen.

Thus, while the previous section called for keeping experiential, on-the-ground training in play for health science students, this section points to the necessity of preparing students for technologically mediated patient care.

Unfortunately, professors may be slow to integrate such lessons into established curriculum. For example, Bedor Hiland's interviews with teletherapists suggest they received little discussion of providing therapy in technologically mediated contexts: "Michelle told me that, during her education, all discussions of teletherapy were limited to the problems it could create" (136). Similarly, research on therapist training has found that graduate programs tend to emphasize traditional career paths for their students, overlooking careers that entail virtual services (Anthony).

However, we might look internationally to countries that are thinking robustly about training providers for digital contexts. For example, Finland has recently been conducting needs analysis for delivering digital services in the health and social care sector. The SotePeda 24/7 project, which ran from 2018 to 2020, aimed to increase "competencies in developing digital services in the health and social care sector, and to create digital pedagogical solutions to support multidisciplinary learning" (Värri et al., "National SotePeda"). Through questionnaires, interviews, and workshops of stakeholders, the project identified digital services competencies and created ready-to-use educational content material (Värri et al., "Definition"). Those materials could serve as a starting point for health educators who are invested in helping their students prepare for virtual or technologically mediated care.

In addition, this book demonstrates that studying technological mediation will continue to be an embodied endeavor. Shifting our attention toward virtual communication does not mean abandoning the material and embodied rhetorical frameworks that have gained traction in rhetorical studies but instead makes them even more relevant. From attending to a "materiality of informatics" (Hayles) that recognizes how bodies are modified to interface with machines to accounting for affective engagement with algorithmic alarms (Bailey et al.), let us keep the body in focus going forward, especially by drawing on fieldwork that integrates the researchers' physical experiences with technological mediation.

Distributions of Power

As my previous discussions have shown, new technological contexts have the potential to both reify gendered and racialized biases as well as transform them. Undoubtedly, we cannot fall into the trap of viewing technologies as neutral apparatuses free from the biases of human intervention (Noble; Benjamin; Barad, *Meeting*). However, the technologies I consider in this book—patient manikins, physical therapy modalities, and virtual patient monitoring—all transform the physical, emotional, and discursive actions of healthcare providers in radical ways. Thus, it is important to attend to both the possibilities and the limitations of these technologies for addressing the needs of marginalized professionals in these fields as well as marginalized patients.

While gender studies scholars have critiqued simulation manikins for their whitewashed, male representation of patient bodies (Sundén; Johnson), I call attention to simulators in intra-action with students, instructors, and the clinical environment. This focus on intra-action still recognizes limitations of the robotic manikin, but it also highlights how lessons about gender and race exist beyond the physical representations of the robot. These lessons emerge through the patient preparation sheet that students receive, the instructor's portrayal of the patient's positionality and concerns, and the student debriefs about patient care. Thus, a complex rhetorical ecology produces lessons about marginalized identities. The troublesome example that I discuss at the end of chapter 2 demonstrates how these multiple factors might come together to reinforce stereotypes and problematic student interventions. However, by bringing individuals from marginalized backgrounds into simulation design and practice (Press) and by constellating possible patient identities during debrief conversations (Barad, *Meeting*), instructors and students can address these limitations. Because the limitations are not only about a single machine's deficiencies, solutions are also distributed and intra-active as well.

In contrast to nursing, which is typically seen as a feminized field, physical therapy has sought to distance itself from a feminized identity to gain professional legitimacy, especially in biomedical contexts (Ottosson; Linker). Similarly, the field has had an ambiguous relationship to technology, since overrelying on technological interventions in patient movement risks reducing PTs' role to technicians rather than scientific experts (Sahrmann). When it came to navigating technological tools in the lab, I found that differing reactions to the new technologies countered students' stereotypes about bodies. Thus, when a macho male student cringed at a low level of electrical stimulation, this was a good reminder for his partner to be attentive to all patients and not to rely on assumptions about how they might respond to care. At the same time, however, as the group giggled at these unexpected reactions and the instructor teased the student, the hidden curriculum in the lab also reinforced gendered views about pain tolerance and the idea that professionalism meant masculine presentation.

Finally, as with many forms of body work, tele-sitting is a racialized and gendered profession; many of the participants in my study were women of color. This work is still clearly marginalized, offering low pay compared with other healthcare roles, with little professional training or support. Chapter 1 elaborates on the various networks of economic exchange that lead to unequal distributions of body work across individuals (Hochschild, *Commercialization*; Yam). At the same time, the virtual context of the VICU created certain affordances for body workers. Participants in my study had the option to use automated recordings to intervene with patients, rather than their own voices, providing an opportunity to mitigate patient stereotypes that might shape their compliance. They also had a great deal of flexibility in their own physical experiences in the VICU—to stand or sit while working or to use weights. And many of them expressed the reduced emotional and physical load of tele-sitting compared with previous hospital work. Their distance from patients enabled them to see themselves in these positions long-term, working part-time to maintain health benefits as a kind of alternative retirement.

This attitude toward work is not one we frequently see among body workers, who often experience a great deal of physical and emotional exhaustion because of their job requirements. In tele-sitting, then, we see potential for women of color to have access to flexible, long-term careers in body work, assuming this work is not further outsourced internationally or to machines. Even better would be to find ways for their voices to become part of official records, so that their patient sense could have a role in improving patient care. This is especially pertinent given the Black maternal health crisis in America and the ongoing call for more Black women physicians (Campbell, "Not Just Doctors").

Rhetorical body work and the concept of patient sense, thus, direct rhetoricians toward new modes of conceptualizing equity in health communication and care. These concepts move us away from pat critiques of technologies that do not perfectly represent human bodies and toward a focus on meaning-making in intra-action. They encourage attention to the hidden curriculum in health science classrooms, where efforts to emphasize expertise and protect professional status might simultaneously devalue certain perspectives or experiences. And they complicate our understanding of what might constitute "good jobs" in healthcare and where individuals from minoritized backgrounds might be able to exert influence in patient care.

My examples also show how both health students and instructors are constantly involved in ethical decision-making, hearkening back to my discussion of phronesis in chapter 1, which recognized it as a praxis tied to scientific knowledge, but also its orientation "toward proper judgment and action" (Smith 93). At times, I think scholars in the humanities run the risk of viewing ourselves as the researchers who are alone invested in ethical teaching and learning (Campbell, "Rhetoric of Health"). I hope the examples in this book help demonstrate otherwise, showing how practitioners in nursing, physical therapy, and tele-observation are equally attentive to the ethical dimensions of teaching patient sense in their fields. In part, this can lead to more scholarly collaboration, as we consider together the kinds of reflective practice that can help students integrate professional and embodied knowledge with an eye toward equity in care.

Overall, this book has called for greater attention to the role of rhetorical body work and patient sense in health practitioner training and practice. In doing so, it pushes back against the age-old dualism that separates mind and body, each of which has been reified at different moments in academic thought—the cultural turn, the discursive turn, the material turn. With the spread of new technologies in healthcare, we can see the real-time risks of such a separation. While we might have expected the robots to take over physical labor (and they have in certain spheres), Topol's optimistic vision of an AI future is one in which automating the rhetorical labor of the physician allows them to be physically and emotionally present with patients once again. By contrast, I point to the need for health practitioners to bring their full selves—mind and body—to technologically mediated patient care. Like Sauer ("Embodied Knowledge" 161) argues, we can work toward two-way communication that brings the intuitive, embodied knowledge of practitioners into exchange with technological information and mediation.

Nursing simulations, physical therapy labs, and virtual care units each offer different visions of how rhetorical body work is maintained and transformed through technological mediation. All point to the ongoing risks of interanimating bodies and technologies in healthcare—reifying stereotypes about patients; reinforcing assumptions about expertise and what "counts" as scientific knowledge; and devaluing practitioners' patient sense and discourse. However, they also offer moments of hope and inspiration. We see a nursing student prompted by a poorly crying manikin who learns to sit with a patient through a difficult moment rather than rush to solutions. We see a physical therapy student who learns to question his assumptions about pain tolerance when his macho classmate cringes during electrical stimulation and we watch him consider how he might communicate about stimulation with a patient who is similarly struggling. We see devalued workers who are often emotionally and physically drained by their body work find a job that they can imagine themselves thriving in long-term.

One question, then, is how to find these moments of potential. In response, I would call rhetoricians toward fieldwork and the study of new health technologies in intra-action, challenging approaches that aim to critique or undermine technologies without attending to them in moments of use. Another question is how to capitalize on these moments to create a new vision for health technologies in the future. Here, rhetoricians can lead the way in challenging versions of a technofuture that devalue rhetorical action—embodied, emotional, and discursive. The lens of rhetorical body work can instead call us to recognize and value the rhetoric in body work and the body in rhetorical work. Thus, we can center the unique patient sense that human bodies bring to healthcare, while not rejecting the advantages that new technologies offer as well.

ACKNOWLEDGMENTS

First and foremost, this book would not have been possible without the generosity of countless instructors, students, and health practitioners who gave both their time and their trust in opening their workplaces to me. While I maintain their anonymity here, I hope that I have done justice to their experiences. I am incredibly grateful for their willingness to collaborate and offer a window into their day-to-day practices and activities.

Thank you to my mentors at the University of Washington, who offered critical insights from the very start of this project. Candice Rai's guidance helped me to recognize the value of rhetorical fieldwork and to enter my research spaces with consideration and care. Her and Anis Bawarshi's feedback strengthened my analytic skills while also giving me confidence in the value of my project and ideas. I am grateful for Gail Stygall's attention to language and gender, which infuse so many of the arguments in this book, and to those who formed my intellectual community at UW, including Alison Cardinal, Roger Chao, Jennifer Eidem, Jacqueline Fiscus-Cannaday, Jennifer LeMesurier, and Misty Anne Winzenried.

I have been so fortunate for collaborations with colleagues and friends as well. Thank you to Elizabeth Angeli for many conversations about intuition in health communication and for being a first reader of this book. What a lucky break to start my academic career with her by my side! Thank you to Elisabeth Miller for her collaboration on pedagogies of empathy in healthcare and for her insights on the publishing process. Thank you to Shion Guha, Amrita George, and Olga Kozlova for helping me to better understand communication and health technology from interdisciplinary perspectives. Thanks to Michelle Smith, Sarah Hallenbeck, and the participants in the Rhetoric Society of America "Material Feminisms and the Rhetoricity of Work" workshop in summer 2023 that enriched my theoretical framing of gender and work. And thank you to the many participants in the Rhetoric of Health and Medicine Symposium and members of the Medical Rhetoric Special Interest Group. They all are truly my intellectual "family," and my work has benefited immensely from their insights and feedback.

Many of my colleagues at Marquette University have helped to ensure that the English department is also an academic home. Thanks to Gerry Canavan, Jenn Fishman, Leah Flack, and Rebecca Nowacek for support and encouragement in the early stages of my career. Thanks to Liza Strakhov and Ben Pladek for their friendship and sage advice. And thanks to Jenna Green for her many contributions to first-year writing that helped ensure this book could get written.

My work has also benefited from financial support at Marquette University and beyond. A Future of Work Pilot Grant from the National Science Foundation in 2021 (Award #2026607) set the groundwork for my study of tele-observers in chapter 4. A Marquette summer research grant in 2021 covered my research time, a video camera, and stipends for participants in chapter 3. Marquette's Institute for Women's Leadership (IWL) provided stipends for research participants in chapter 4 in summer 2022. Marquette's Summer Research Institute also offered financial and emotional support to get back into writing in summer 2022. Finally, the IWL provided subvention funds toward publication of this book.

Excerpts from chapters 1 and 2 of the book appeared in my article titled "Rhetorical Body Work: Professional Embodiment in Health Provider Education and the Technical Writing Classroom" in *Technical Communication Quarterly,* © 2020 Association of Teachers of Technical Writing (ATTW). I am grateful to Taylor & Francis (https://www.tandfonline.com) on behalf of ATTW for their permission to reprint portions of the article. Thank you also to Bellin College and the Center for Nursing Philosophy at University of California–Irvine for the opportunity to share this work-in-progress and receive feedback from their communities.

Thank you to the editorial team at The Ohio State University Press and editors of the New Directions in Rhetoric and Materiality series for championing this book. From our first conversation, I felt that Taralee Cyphers shared my vision for the book, and it has been strengthened by her thoughtful feedback throughout the process. Thanks also to the anonymous reviewers who offered their insights with care and kindness; the book is better because of them.

My local community, friends, and family supported this project in many ways—from thoughtful conversations to fun distractions to childcare. Thank you to Barre Milwaukee, especially Christina and Annie, for ensuring that I continued to care for my own body during the writing of this book. Thanks to the COA Youth & Family Centers for creating a space for parents to build community in our neighborhood and to all the childcare providers, friends, and family who helped care for my daughter to make the writing possible. Thanks to Mary Little and Ashley Jones for cross-country visits, long-distance video chats, and endless encouragement.

Thanks to my mom, Suzanne Campbell, for introducing me to nursing simulations and modeling what it looks like to balance career and family. Thanks also to my dad, Gerard Campbell, and my brother, Gregory Campbell. They all have always taken my work seriously and been my greatest champions; I am so grateful for that support. To my family-in-law—Corinne Dempsey, Nick Garigliano, Sam Garigliano, Libby Rosa, and Julia Fillman—how did I get so lucky? They all bring so much joy and love to my life, and their influence on this book shows up in big and small ways.

Finally, thanks to my partner, Jack Garigliano, and daughter, Vera Garigliano. This project has been as much a part of Jack's life as it has mine for the last decade. His humor, compassion, and teamwork made it all possible. And to Vera, the future dancer or scientist or singer or doctor or mom or teacher, et cetera, thanks for helping keep me in the moment and reminding me of all the good all around me. I hope that whatever she chooses for her future career, she gets to experience real moments of human connection across bodies and space. In short, this book is an argument for continuing to value that kind of work.

APPENDIX 1

Nursing Simulation Interview Questions

First-Round Interview

General Background

- Can you tell me a little bit about yourself?
    - Where did you grow up? What do your parents do?
    - What were your strengths as a student growing up? What were your weaknesses?
- Why did you decide to study nursing in college?
    - What appeals to you about being a nurse?
    - Did you know anyone who was a nurse growing up? If so, what did you learn from this person about the field of nursing?
- Why did you choose to attend [X University] to study nursing? What appealed to you about their program?

Coursework So Far

- What courses have you taken in the School of Nursing so far?
    - What have you learned that will help you the most to be a successful nurse?
    - What has been most challenging about your nursing courses so far?
- What kinds of writing have you been doing in your nursing courses?

- What do you think are the goals of those writing assignments?
- How might writing assignments be different this year?
  - What are you looking forward (or hoping) to learn this coming year?
    - What questions or concerns do you have about those topics right now?

Understanding of the Field

- What do you think are the 3–4 most important traits to have as a nurse? Why?
- What kinds of communication strategies do you see as most important to nurses? Why?
- What kinds of writing do you imagine having to do as a nurse? When will it be important?
  - Does any of the writing in your classes seem relevant to this future writing?
- What would it mean to you to embody a nursing identity? What kinds of physical movements, gestures or actions are most fundamental to nursing practice?
  - How does a nurse carry his or herself or handle patients? How do nurses move?
- How would you describe the field of nursing's orientation towards patients? What about towards others in the hospital or clinic (doctors, assistants, other nurses, etc.)?
  - What feels unique about a nurse's orientation to others in clinical practice?
  - What do you like about this perspective? What don't you like about it?
  - In what ways have your nursing courses been teaching this orientation?
- What do you see as some of the biggest challenges facing nurses today?
  - What kinds of skills will be most important for them to face those challenges?

Simulation Follow-Up Interviews (×3)

General Background

- In your understanding, what were the learning goals of this particular simulation?
    - What connections did you see between what you're learning in class or in your clinical placement and the learning goals of the simulation?
- Can you tell me a little bit about your experience with the simulation in general?
    - What felt like it went well to you? What didn't?
    - What did you learn from your own simulation and from watching your peers?
    - If you were to do the simulation again, what would you do differently?

Discursive Learning

- What did you learn about nursing "talk" or writing from this simulation?
- What strategies did you use to communicate with the simulator during the scenario?
    - What worked well about your communication?
    - What would you do differently in the future?
    - What did you learn from watching peers communicate with the simulator?
- What strategies did you use to communicate with your peers during the scenario?
    - [Repeat sub-questions above]
- Do you see connections between what you learned about nursing talk in the scenario and the writing you're doing in your nursing classes or clinical placements?
- Do you see yourself using what you've learning about communication from this scenario in the future? In what ways?

Embodied Learning

- What did you learn about the physical movements, gestures or actions of nursing from this simulation?
- In what ways did you physically interact with the simulator during the scenario?
    - What worked well about that interaction?
    - What would you do differently in the future?
    - What did you learn from watching peers physically interact with the simulator?
- In what ways did you physically interact with your peers during the scenario?
    - [Repeat sub-questions above]
- Do you see yourself using what you've learning about the physical movements, actions, or gestures of nursing from this scenario in the future? In what ways?

Relational Learning

- What did you learn about nurse's orientations towards patients and others in the hospital or clinic (doctors, assistants, other nurses, etc.) from this simulation?
- What was your attitude towards the patient (simulator) during the scenario? Why?
    - Do you feel that it was the right attitude/orientation to have? Why or why not?
    - Do you think you would feel differently towards a patient with in a similar situation in the future? Why or why not?
    - What did you learn from watching peers' attitudes towards the simulator?
- What was your attitude towards your peers during the scenario? Why?
    - [Repeat sub-questions above]
- Do you see yourself using what you've learning about nurse's orientations towards patients and others from this scenario in the future? In what ways?

APPENDIX 2

Physical Therapy Interview Questions

First-Round Interview

General Background

- For demographic context, can you please tell me how you identify in terms of gender, race, and/or ethnicity? For example, I identify as a white female.
- Why did you decide to study Physical Therapy?
    - Direct admit or transfer student?
    - Have you had any clinical experiences so far?
- What have you learned in your classes and/or clinical experiences so far about writing or communication as a physical therapist?
- How do you see the Physical Technologies class fitting into your PT curriculum? What is the role/purpose of this class?
- What are you hoping to learn about writing or communication in this course?
    - What can be learned from practicing on classmates and what can't be?

Understanding of the Field

- When you imagine your day-to-day work as a future PT, what kinds of writing and communication will be most central?

- How would you describe the field of PT's orientation towards patients? What about towards others in the hospital or clinic (doctors, assistants, nurses, etc.)?
  - What are some strategies for good interprofessional communication?
- What do you see as some of the biggest challenges facing PTs today?

Follow-Up Interview

Learning in the Course

- How did the final practical for the course go?
  - What went well? What do you wish had gone differently?
  - Do you feel like you were able to demonstrate what you've learned?
- What are some of your biggest take-aways from the course in terms of **skills/techniques**?
  - What do you think will be similar when you use these skills in clinical contexts? What will be different?
- What were some of your biggest take-aways in terms of **writing or communication**?
  - What do you think will be similar when you use these skills in clinical contexts? What will be different?
- What do you see yourself using the most?
- Overall, how would you describe your experience with the course? Anything else you want me to know about your learning in this course?

Looking at the Clip

- Can you describe for me what's happening in this clip?
  - What were the main learning goals of this particular lab?
  - What aspect of the lab are you focused on here and why?
- What **skills/techniques** are you demonstrating in this clip?
  - How will these be similar in clinical contexts? How will they be different?
  - What went well and what would you do differently next time?
- What **communication** strategies are you demonstrating in this clip?

- How will these be similar in clinical contexts? How will they be different?
- What went well and what would you differently next time?
- What did this feel like for you? How would describe it?
  - Anything else you noticed?

Looking at the SOAP Notes

- Can you give me some context on this note?
  - What lab were they associated with?
  - How much guidance were you given?
- How does this note compare to other ones written for this class? What about for ones you've written in other classes?
- What went well while writing this note?

APPENDIX 3

Tele-Observation Interview Questions

Only Interview

Background

- For demographic context, can you please tell me how you identify in terms of gender, race, and/or ethnicity? For example, I identify as a white female.
- Can you tell me a little bit about yourself?
    - How long have you been working in the VICU?
    - What interested you about the position?
- What kind of education did you receive prior to starting the tele-op position?
    - How does that training inform your current work?
    - What kinds of lessons do you find yourself drawing on the most?
    - What kinds of lessons feel the least useful looking back?
    - What kinds of embodied training did you receive? How does that inform your work in tele-ops?
    - Were there things you wish had been emphasized in your program that weren't?
- Did you have any prior work experience in healthcare?
    - How did that experience inform your current work?
    - What kinds of experiences from previous work do you find yourself drawing on the most?
    - Any embodied learning in the workplace that informs your work in tele-ops?

- What kinds of training did you receive from the hospital before starting at the VICU?
    - How does that training inform your current work?
    - What kinds of lessons do you find yourself drawing on the most?
    - What kinds of lessons feel the least useful looking back?
    - Were there things you wish had been emphasized in your program that weren't?
- How do you explain to family members or friends what you do?
    - What do you like best about your job? What do you like least?
    - Would you recommend this job to others? Why or why not?
- What are your future educational/career goals?
    - How do you see the tele-ops position fitting into those goals?
    - What do you think will be most useful from this experience going forward?

VICU Experiences

- Could you describe a typical day in your current job?
    - What are typical workday activities?
    - How is time divided between these activities?
- What strategies do you use to manage the large number of patients you are observing?
    - How do you decide which patients to prioritize?
    - What might cause you to change your priorities?
    - Are there instances where you've missed something important? What happened?

Communication

- What kinds of communication do you do with patients on a day-to-day basis?
    - What kinds of actions will cause you to speak over the mic?
    - What strategies do you use to communicate with difficult patients?
- What kinds of documentation are required when you take different actions?

- What kinds of communication with other providers do you do on a day-to-day basis?
    - With other tele-ops? With VICU RN's? With RN's and physicians on the floor?
    - Where do you feel like there are communication troubles across specialties?
- Can you walk me through a scenario with a hypothetical patient that shows the different kinds of communication practices you use? (ie if you had a patient that needed interventions, what would you do first, second, third, when would you document, etc.)

Embodied Practices

- What is your physical experience like working in the VICU?
    - Does it tax one part of your body more than others?
    - How does this compare to your physical experience of other healthcare workplaces?
    - Do you see yourself being able to perform this work long-term? Why or why not?
- What is your emotional experience like working in the VICU?
    - Is it stressful? Boring? Do you feel calm or on edge?
    - How does this compare to your emotional experience of other healthcare workplaces?
- What bodily moves are you watching for in your patients?
    - How do you differentiate between problematic and okay moves?
    - Are there times when you've gotten this wrong or overlooked something important?
- What emotional states are you looking for in your patients?
    - What clues do you look for to cue those states?
    - Are there times when you've gotten this wrong or overlooked something important?
- Can you think of a time when you wished you were physically in the room with the patient?
    - What physical actions would have taken? What did you do instead?
    - What would have been different if you were physically present with them?

WORKS CITED

Acker, Joan. "Hierarchies, Jobs, Bodies: A Theory of Gendered Organizations." *Gender & Society* 4, no. 2, 1990, pp. 139–58, https://doi.org/10.1177/089124390004002002.

Allen, Caitlin Burns. *You Don't Look Sick: Epistemic Injustice, Ethos, and Embodied Expertise in Narratives of Chronic Illness.* 2004. U of Louisville, PhD dissertation.

Angeli, Elizabeth L. *Rhetorical Work in Emergency Medical Services: Communicating in the Unpredictable Workplace.* Routledge, 2018.

Angeli, Elizabeth, and Lillian Campbell. "Designing 'Writing for Health and Medicine': Course Arcs, Anchors, and Action." *Programmatic Perspectives* 14, no. 1, 2023, pp. 165–74.

Angeli, Elizabeth L., and Lillian Campbell. "Intuition in Healthcare Communication Practices: Initial Findings from a Qualitative Inquiry." *2017 IEEE International Professional Communication Conference Proceedings.* IEEE, 2017, pp. 1–6, https://doi.org/10.1109/IPCC.2017.8013931.

Anthony, Kate. "Training Therapists to Work Effectively Online and Offline within Digital Culture." *British Journal of Guidance & Counselling* 43, no. 1, 2015, pp. 36–42, https://doi.org/10.1080/03069885.2014.924617.

Arduser, Lora. *Living Chronic: Agency and Expertise in the Rhetoric of Diabetes.* The Ohio State UP, 2017.

Arendt, Hannah. "Labor, Work, Action." *Amor Mundi: Explorations in the Faith and Thought of Hannah Arendt,* edited by James W. Bernauer, Springer Netherlands, 1987, pp. 29–42.

Ariail, Jennie, and Thomas G. Smith. "Concept Analysis: Using an Academic Nursing Genre for Writing Instruction in Nursing." *Rhetoric of Healthcare: Essays toward a New Disciplinary Inquiry,* edited by Barbara Heufferon and Stuart C. Brown, Hampton, 2008, pp. 243–63.

Bailey, Thomas C., et al. "A Trial of a Real-Time Alert for Clinical Deterioration in Patients Hospitalized on General Medical Wards: Deterioration Alerts on Medical Wards." *Journal of Hospital Medicine* 8, no. 5, 2013, pp. 236–42, https://doi.org/10.1002/jhm.2009.

Bannow, Tara. "Med School Changes Pelvic Exam Instruction." *Minnesota Daily,* 17 Feb. 2010, https://mndaily.com/205482/uncategorized/med-school-changes-pelvic-exam-instruction/.

Barad, Karen. *Meeting the Universe Halfway: Quantum Physics and the Entanglement of Matter and Meaning.* Duke UP, 2007.

Barad, Karen. "Posthumanist Performativity: Toward an Understanding of How Matter Comes to Matter." *Signs: Journal of Women in Culture and Society* 28, no. 3, 2003, pp. 801–31, https://doi.org/10.1086/345321.

Bas-Sarmiento, Pilar, et al. "Empathy Training in Health Sciences: A Systematic Review." *Nurse Education in Practice* 44, 2020, article 102739, https://doi.org/10.1016/j.nepr.2020.102739.

Bawarshi, Anis. *Genre and the Invention of the Writer: Reconsidering the Place of Invention in Composition.* Utah State UP, 2003.

Bazerman, Charles. *Shaping Written Knowledge: Genre and Activity of Experimental Article in Science.* U of Wisconsin P, 1989.

Bedor Hiland, Emma. *Therapy Tech: The Digital Transformation of Mental Healthcare.* U of Minnesota P, 2021.

Bennett, Jane. *Vibrant Matter: A Political Ecology of Things.* Duke UP, 2010.

Bennett, Jeffrey A. *Managing Diabetes: The Cultural Politics of Disease.* New York UP, 2019.

Benjamin, Ruha. *Race After Technology: Abolitionist Tools for the New Jim Code.* Polity, 2019.

Blankenship, Lisa. *Changing the Subject: A Theory of Rhetorical Empathy.* UP Colorado, 2019.

Bloom-Pojar, Rachel. *Translanguaging Outside the Academy: Negotiating Rhetoric and Healthcare in the Spanish Caribbean.* National Council of the Teachers of English, 2018.

Bourdieu, Pierre. "Outline of a Theory of Practice." *The New Social Theory Reader,* edited by Jeffrey C. Alexander and Steven Seidman, Routledge, 2020, pp. 80–86.

Breen, Gerald-Mark, and Jonathan Matusitz. "An Evolutionary Examination of Telemedicine: A Health and Computer-Mediated Communication Perspective." *Social Work in Public Health* 25, no. 1, 2010, pp. 59–71.

Britt, Elizabeth C. *Reimagining Advocacy: Rhetorical Education in the Legal Clinic.* Pennsylvania State UP, 2018.

Brittenham, Rebecca. "The Interference Narrative and the Real Value of Student Work." *College Composition and Communication* 68, no. 3, 2017, pp. 526–58.

Brown, Patrick R., et al. "Actions Speak Louder Than Words: The Embodiment of Trust by Healthcare Professionals in Gynaeoncology." *Sociology of Health & Illness* 33, no. 2, 2011, pp. 280–95.

Butler, Rachel, et al. "Estimating Time Physicians and Other Health Care Workers Spend with Patients in an Intensive Care Unit Using a Sensor Network." *American Journal of Medicine* 131, no. 8, 2018, pp. 972–79. https://doi.org/10.1016/j.amjmed.2018.03.015.

Campbell, Lillian. "Not Just Doctors: Woman-Dominated Health Work as a Site for Rhetorical Research and Professional Change." *Peitho* 26, no. 2, 2024, pp. 105–18.

Campbell, Lillian. "The Rhetoric of Health and Medicine as a 'Teaching Subject': Lessons from the Medical Humanities and Simulation Pedagogy." *Technical Communication Quarterly* 27, no. 1, 2018, pp. 7–20, https://doi.org/10.1080/10572252.2018.1401348.

Campbell, Lillian. "Simulating Gender: Student Learning in Clinical Nursing Simulations." *Interrogating Gendered Pathologies,* edited by Erin Clark and Michelle Eble, Utah State UP, 2020, pp. 83–100.

Campbell, Lillian. *Simulating Nursing: Rhetoric, Materiality, and Disciplinary Learning.* 2016. U of Washington, PhD dissertation.

Campbell, Lillian. "Simulation Genres and Student Uptake: The Patient Health Record in Clinical Nursing Simulations." *Written Communication* 34, no. 3, 2017, pp. 255–79, https://doi.org/10.1177/0741088317716413.

Campbell, Lillian, and Elizabeth L. Angeli. "Embodied Healthcare Intuition: A Taxonomy of Sensory Cues Used by Healthcare Providers." *Rhetoric of Health & Medicine* 2, no. 4, 2019, pp. 353–83, https://doi.org/10.5744/rhm.2019.1017.

Campbell, Lillian, and Jaclyn Fiscus-Cannaday. "Multimodal Analysis and the Composition TAship." *Standing at the Threshold: Working Through Liminality in the Composition and Rhetoric TAship*, edited by William Macauley, Utah State UP, 2021, pp. 31–59.

Campbell, Lillian, and Elisabeth L. Miller. "Pedagogies of Rhetorical Empathy-in-Action: Role Playing and Story Sharing in Healthcare Education." *Rhetoric of Health & Medicine* 6, no. 1, 2023, pp. 36–63.

Campbell, Lillian, et al. "Practitioner Attitudes Towards an Early Warning System: From Professional Distraction to Relational Support." *2021 IEEE International Professional Communication Conference Proceedings*. IEEE, 2021, pp. 123–24, https://doi.org/10.1109/ProComm52174.2021.00028.

Chávez, Karma R. "The Body: An Abstract and Actual Rhetorical Concept." *Rhetoric Society Quarterly* 48, no. 3, 2018, pp. 242–50, https://doi.org/10.1080/02773945.2018.1454182.

Clayson, Ashley. "Distributed Writing as a Lens for Examining Writing as Embodied Practice." *Technical Communication Quarterly* 27, no. 3, 2018, pp. 217–26, https://doi.org/10.1080/10572252.2018.1479607.

Coffey, Julia. "Bodies, Body Work and Gender: Exploring a Deleuzian Approach." *Journal of Gender Studies* 22, no. 1, 2013, pp. 3–16, https://doi.org/10.1080/09589236.2012.714076.

Cooper, Simon, et al. "Managing Deteriorating Patients: Registered Nurses' Performance in a Simulated Setting." *Open Nursing Journal* 5, no. 1, 2011, pp. 120–26, https://doi.org/10.2174/1874434601105010120.

Crocco, Francesco. "Simulating Utopia: Critical Simulation and the Teaching of Utopia." *Journal of Interactive Technology and Pedagogy* 7, 2015, https://cuny.manifoldapp.org/read/simulating-utopia-critical-simulation-and-the-teaching-of-utopia-1611526c-ef17-4cfa-9870-e9314f7033d3/section/a8d3100b-9963-4293-8a12-76241680aa35.

Cushman, Jeremy. "Distributed Labor, Writing, and an Automotive Repair Shop." *Literacy in Practice: Writing in Private, Public, and Working Lives*, edited by Patrick Thomas and Pamela Takayoshi, Routledge, 2015, pp. 217–29.

Davis, Janet, et al. "A Comparative Study of Patient Sitters with Video Monitoring versus In-Room Sitters." *Journal of Nursing Education and Practice* 7, no. 3, 2017, pp. 137–42, https://doi.org/10.5430/jnep.v7n3p137.

Dearing, Karen S., and Sheryl Steadman. "Enhancing Intellectual Empathy: The Lived Experience of Voice Simulation." *Perspectives in Psychiatric Care* 45, no. 3, 2009, pp. 173–82, https://doi.org/10.1111/j.1744-6163.2009.00219.x.

Derkatch, Colleen. *Bounding Biomedicine: Evidence and Rhetoric in the New Science of Alternative Medicine*. U of Chicago P, 2019.

DeStigter, Todd. "Public Displays of Affection: Political Community through Critical Empathy." *Research in the Teaching of English* 33, no. 3, 1999, pp. 235–44.

Detweiler, Jane, and Claudia Peyton. "Defining Occupations: A Chronotopic Study of Narrative Genres in a Health Discipline's Emergence." *Written Communication* 16, no. 4, 1999, pp. 412–68, https://doi.org/10.1177/0741088399016004002.

Dolmage, Jay. "Metis, Mêtis, Mestiza, Medusa: Rhetorical Bodies across Rhetorical Traditions." *Rhetoric Review* 28, no. 1, 2009, pp. 1–28, https://doi.org/10.1080/07350190802540690.

Egenes, Karen. "History of Nursing." *Issues and Trends in Nursing: Essential Knowledge for Today and Tomorrow*, edited by Gayle Roux and Judith A. Halstead, Jones and Bartlett Learning LLC, 2009, pp. 1–26.

Federici, Silvia. *Revolution at Point Zero: Housework, Reproduction, and Feminist Struggle*. PM Press, 2020.

Fisher, Murray J. "'Being a Chameleon': Labour Processes of Male Nurses Performing Bodywork." *Journal of Advanced Nursing* 65, no. 12, 2009, pp. 2668–77, https://doi.org/10.1111/j.1365-2648.2009.05120.x.

Florea, Mona, et al. "Using an Information Literacy Program to Prepare Nursing Students to Practice in a Virtual Workplace." *Handbook of Research on Virtual Workplaces and the New Nature of Business Practices*, edited by Pavel Zemliansky and Kirk St. Amant, IGI Global, 2008, pp. 317–33.

Foley, Claire, and Maura Dowling. "How Do Nurses Use the Early Warning Score in Their Practice? A Case Study from an Acute Medical Unit." *Journal of Clinical Nursing* 28, no. 7–8, 2019, pp. 1183–92, https://doi.org/10.1111/jocn.14713.

Foucault, Michel. *The Birth of the Clinic*. Routledge, 2002.

Fountain, T. Kenny. *Rhetoric in the Flesh: Trained Vision, Technical Expertise, and the Gross Anatomy Lab*. Routledge, 2014.

Fraser, Nancy. "Behind Marx's Hidden Abode: For an Expanded Conception of Capitalism." *New Left Review* 86, Mar.–Apr. 2014, pp. 55–72.

Frost, Erin A. "Apparent Feminism as a Methodology for Technical Communication and Rhetoric." *Journal of Business and Technical Communication* 30, no. 1, 2016, pp. 3–28, https://doi.org/10.1177/1050651915602295.

Gawande, Atul. "Why Doctors Hate Their Computers." *New Yorker* 12 (2018), https://www.newyorker.com/magazine/2018/11/12/why-doctors-hate-their-computers.

George, Gerard, et al. "Big Data and Management." *Academy of Management Journal* 57, no. 2, 2014, pp. 321–26, https://doi.org/10.5465/amj.2014.4002.

George, Molly. "Interactions in Expert Service Work: Demonstrating Professionalism in Personal Training." *Journal of Contemporary Ethnography* 37, no. 1, 2008, pp. 108–31.

Gieryn, Thomas F. "Boundary-Work and the Demarcation of Science from Non-Science: Strains and Interests in Professional Ideologies of Scientists." *American Sociological Review* 48, no. 6, 1983, pp. 781–95, https://doi.org/10.2307/2095325.

Gimlin, Debra. *Body Work: Beauty and Self-Image in American Culture*. U of California P, 2002.

Gimlin, Debra. "What Is 'Body Work'? A Review of the Literature." *Sociology Compass* 1, no. 1, 2007, pp. 353–70, https://doi.org/10.1111/j.1751-9020.2007.00015.x.

Gold, David, and Jessica Enoch, editors. *Women at Work: Rhetorics of Gender and Labor*. U of Pittsburgh P, 2019.

Graham, S. Scott. *The Doctor and the Algorithm: Promise, Peril, and the Future of Health AI*. Oxford UP, 2022.

Haas, Christina, and Stephen P. Witte. "Writing as an Embodied Practice: The Case of Engineering Standards." *Journal of Business and Technical Communication* 15, no. 4, 2001, pp. 413–57, https://doi.org/10.1177/105065190101500402.

Hafferty, Fredric W., and Ronald Franks. "The Hidden Curriculum, Ethics Teaching, and the Structure of Medical Education." *Academic Medicine* 69, no. 11, 1994, pp. 861–71, https://doi.org/10.1097/00001888-199411000-00001.

Halasa-Rappel, Yara A., et al. "Broken Smiles: The Impact of Untreated Dental Caries and Missing Anterior Teeth on Employment." *Journal of Public Health Dentistry* 79, no. 3, 2019, pp. 231–37, https://doi.org/10.1111/jphd.12317.

Hallenbeck, Sarah, and Michelle Smith. "Mapping Topoi in the Rhetorical Gendering of Work." *Peitho* 17, no. 2, 2015, pp. 200–225.

Haraway, Donna. "A Manifesto for Cyborgs: Science, Technology, and Socialist Feminism in the 1980s." *Feminisms*, edited by Sandra Kemp and Judith Squires, Oxford UP, 1998, pp. 474–81.

Harris, Anna. "In a Moment of Mismatch: Overseas Doctors' Adjustments in New Hospital Environments." *Sociology of Health & Illness* 33, no. 2, 2011, pp. 308–20, https://doi.org/10.1111/j.1467-9566.2010.01307.x.

Hawhee, Debra. *Bodily Arts: Rhetoric and Athletics in Ancient Greece*. U of Texas P, 2005.

Hawhee, Debra. *Moving Bodies: Kenneth Burke at the Edges of Language*. U of South Carolina P, 2009.

Hayles, N. Katherine. "The Materiality of Informatics." *Configurations* 1, no. 1, 1993, pp. 147–70, https://doi.org/10.1353/con.1993.0003.

Hertel, John Paul, and Barbara Millis. *Using Simulations to Promote Learning in Higher Education*. Stylus Publishing, 2002.

Hochschild, Arlie Russell. *The Commercialization of Intimate Life: Notes from Home and Work*. U of California P, 2003.

Hochschild, Arlie Russell. *The Managed Heart: Commercialization of Human Feeling*. U of California P, 1983.

Holzinger, Andreas, et al. "Causability and Explainability of Artificial Intelligence in Medicine." *Wiley Interdisciplinary Reviews: Data Mining and Knowledge Discovery* 9, no. 4, 2019, article e1312, https://doi.org/10.1002/widm.1312.

Ivinson, Gabrielle, and Emma Renold. "Writing as Bodywork: Poverty, Literacy and Unspoken Pain in Ex-mining South Wales Valleys Communities." *Resisting Educational Inequality: Reframing Policy and Practice in Schools Serving Vulnerable Communities,* edited by Susanne Gannon, et al., Routledge, 2018, pp. 277–93.

Jack, Jordynn. *Science on the Home Front: American Women Scientists in World War II*. U of Illinois P, 2009.

Jamison, Leslie. *The Empathy Exams: Essays*. Graywolf Press, 2014.

Johnson, Ericka. "The Ghost of Anatomies Past: Simulating the One-Sex Body in Modern Medical Training." *Feminist Theory* 6, no. 2, 2005, pp. 141–59, https://doi.org/10.1177/146470010505369.

Jung, Julie, editor. *Feminist Rhetorical Science Studies: Human Bodies, Posthumanist Worlds*. Southern Illinois UP, 2017.

Kerschbaum, Stephanie L. "Avoiding the Difference Fixation: Identity Categories, Markers of Difference, and the Teaching of Writing." *College Composition and Communication* 63, no. 4, 2012, pp. 616–44.

Kessler, Molly Margaret. *Stigma Stories: Rhetoric, Lived Experience, and Chronic Illness*. The Ohio State UP, 2022.

Kesti, Julie. "Plastic Pelvises Do Not Prepare Doctors for Real Ones." *Minnesota Daily,* 17 Feb. 2010, https://mndaily.com/188968/uncategorized/plastic-pelvises-do-not-prepare-doctors-real-ones.

Knoblauch, A. Abby. "Bodies of Knowledge: Definitions, Delineations, and Implications of Embodied Writing in the Academy." *Composition Studies* 40, no. 2, 2012, pp. 50–65.

Knoblauch, A. Abby, and Marie E. Moeller, editors. *Bodies of Knowledge: Embodied Rhetorics in Theory and Practice*. UP of Colorado, 2022.

Kohn, Linda T., et al. *To Err Is Human: Building a Safer Health System*. National Academy Press, 2000.

Kopelson, Karen. "Rhetoric on the Edge of Cunning; Or, the Performance of Neutrality (Re)Considered as a Composition Pedagogy for Student Resistance." *College Composition & Communication* 55, no. 1, 2003, pp. 115–46, https://www.jstor.org/stable/3594203.

Krasniansky, Adriana. "TeleSitters Are Entering Hospital Rooms: How Will They Change Patient Care?" *Harvard Law: Bill of Health,* 10 Mar. 2020, https://blog.petrieflom.law.harvard.edu/2020/03/10/telesitters-are-entering-hospital-rooms-how-will-they-change-patient-care/.

Kulbaga, Theresa A. "Pleasurable Pedagogies: Reading 'Lolita in Tehran' and the Rhetoric of Empathy." *College English* 70, no. 5, 2008, pp. 506–21.

Lagman, Eileen. "Moving Labor: Transnational Migrant Workers and Affective Literacies of Care." *Literacy in Composition Studies* 3, no. 3, 2015, pp. 1–24, https://doi.org/10.21623/1.3.3.2.

Lång, Kristina, et al. "Artificial Intelligence-Supported Screen Reading versus Standard Double Reading in the Mammography Screening with Artificial Intelligence trial (MASAI): A Clinical Safety Analysis of a Randomised, Controlled, Non-inferiority, Single-Blinded, Screening Accuracy Study." *Lancet Oncology* 24, no. 8, 2023, pp. 936–44, https://doi.org/10.1016/S1470-2045(23)00298-X.

Lapum, Jennifer, et al. "A Cyborg Ontology in Health Care: Traversing into the Liminal Space between Technology and Person-Centred Practice: A Cyborg Ontology." *Nursing Philosophy: An International Journal for Healthcare Professionals* 13, no. 4, 2012, pp. 276–88, https://doi.org/10.1111/j.1466-769X.2012.00543.x.

Latour, Bruno, and Steve Woolgar. *Laboratory Life: The Construction of Scientific Facts.* Princeton UP, 1986.

Lawler, Jocalyn. *Behind the Screens: Nursing, Somology and the Problem of the Body.* Sydney UP, 2006.

Leake, Eric. "Writing Pedagogies of Empathy: As Rhetoric and Disposition." *Composition Forum* 24, 2016, https://compositionforum.com/issue/34/empathy.php.

LeMesurier, Jennifer Lin. "Mobile Bodies: Triggering Bodily Uptake through Movement." *College Composition and Communication* 68, no. 2, 2016, pp. 292–316, https://www.jstor.org/stable/44783563.

LeMesurier, Jennifer Lin. "Somatic Metaphors: Embodied Recognition of Rhetorical Opportunities." *Rhetoric Review* 33, no. 4, 2014, pp. 362–80, https://doi.org/10.1080/07350198.2014.946868.

LeMesurier, Jennifer Lin. "Winking at Excess: Racist Kinesiologies in Childish Gambino's 'This Is America.'" *Rhetoric Society Quarterly* 50, no. 2, 2020, pp. 139–51, https://doi.org/10.1080/02773945.2020.1725615.

Lindquist, Julie. "Class Affects, Classroom Affectations: Working through the Paradoxes of Strategic Empathy." *College English* 67, no. 2, 2004, pp. 187–209, https://doi.org/10.2307/4140717.

Linker, Beth. "Strength and Science: Gender, Physiotherapy, and Medicine in the United States, 1918–35." *Journal of Women's History* 17, no. 3, 2005, pp. 106–32, https://doi.org/10.1353/jowh.2005.0034.

Lu, Min-Zhan, and Bruce Horner. "Composing in a Global-Local Context: Careers, Mobility, Skills." *College English* 72, no. 2, 2009, pp. 113–33.

Macaulay, Thomas. "Flawed Algorithm Used to Determine U.K. Welfare Payments Is 'Pushing People into Poverty.'" *Communications of the ACM,* 2020, https://acmwebvm01.acm.org/news/247831-flawed-algorithm-used-to-determine-uk-welfare-payments-is-pushing-people-into-poverty/fulltext.

Mackiewicz, Jo. *Welding Technical Communication: Teaching and Learning Embodied Knowledge.* State U of New York P, 2022.

Madison, D. Soyini. "Staging Fieldwork/Performing Human Rights." *The SAGE Handbook of Performance Studies,* SAGE Publications, Inc., 2006, pp. 397–418.

Magelssen, Scott. *Simming: Participatory Performance and the Making of Meaning.* U of Michigan P, 2014.

Marotta, Calley. "Who Has the Right to Write? Custodian Writing and White Property in the University." *College English* 81, no. 3, 2019, pp. 163–82, https://www.jstor.org/stable/10.2307/26773421.

Måseide, Per. "Body Work in Respiratory Physiological Examinations." *Sociology of Health & Illness* 33, no. 2, 2011, pp. 296–307, https://doi.org/10.1111/j.1467-9566.2010.01292.x.

Middleton, Michael K., et al. "Articulating Rhetorical Field Methods: Challenges and Tensions." *Western Journal of Communication* 75, no. 4, 2011, pp. 386–406, https://doi.org/10.1080/10570314.2011.586969.

Moeckli, Jane, et al. "Staff Acceptance of a Telemedicine Intensive Care Unit Program: A Qualitative Study." *Journal of Critical Care* 28, no. 6, 2013, pp. 890–901, https://doi.org/10.1016/j.jcrc.2013.05.008.

Moffat, Marilyn. "The History of Physical Therapy Practice in the United States." *Journal of Physical Therapy Education* 17, no. 3, 2003, pp. 15–25, https://doi.org/10.1097/00001416-200310000-00003.

Montgomery, Kathryn. *How Doctors Think: Clinical Judgment and the Practice of Medicine.* Oxford: Oxford UP, 2005.

Morris, Kerri K. "Women and Bladder Cancer: Listening Rhetorically to Healthcare Disparities." *Interrogating Gendered Pathologies,* edited by Erin Clark and Michelle Eble, Utah State UP, 2020, pp. 157–70.

Mulla, Sameena. *The Violence of Care: Rape Victims, Forensic Nurses, and Sexual Assault Intervention.* New York UP, 2014.

Nehring, Wendy M., and Felissa R. Lashley. "Nursing Simulation: A Review of the Past 40 Years." *Simulation & Gaming* 40, no. 4, 2009, pp. 528–52, https://doi.org/10.1177/1046878109332282.

Neumann, Donald A. "Polio: Its Impact on the People of the United States and the Emerging Profession of Physical Therapy." *Journal of Orthopaedic and Sports Physical Therapy* 34, no. 8, 2004, pp. 479–92, https://doi.org/10.2519/jospt.2004.0301.

Noble, Sofiya Umoja. *Algorithms of Oppression: How Search Engines Reinforce Racism.* New York UP, 2018.

Norris, Meriel, and Emma Wainwright. "Learning Professional Touch: An Exploration of Pre-Registration Physiotherapy Students' Experiences." *Physiotherapy Theory and Practice* 38, no. 1, 2022, pp. 90–100, https://doi.org/10.1080/09593985.2020.1725944.

Norris, Sigrid. *Analyzing Multimodal Interaction: A Methodological Framework.* Routledge, 2004.

Opel, Dawn S., and William Hart-Davidson. "The Primary Care Clinic as Writing Space." *Written Communication* 36, no. 3, 2019, pp. 348–78, https://doi.org/10.1177/0741088319839968.

Osorio, Ruth. "Rewriting Maternal Bodies on the Senate Floor." *Bodies of Knowledge: Embodied Rhetorics in Theory and Practice,* edited by Abby A. Knoblauch and Marie E. Moeller, UP of Colorado, 2022, pp. 143–60.

Ottosson, Anders. "Androphobia, Demasculinization, and Professional Conflicts: The Herstories of the Physical Therapy Profession Deconstructed." *Social Science History* 40, no. 3, 2016, pp. 433–61, https://doi.org/10.1017/ssh.2016.13.

Pope-Ruark, Rebecca. "A Case for Metic Intelligence in Technical and Professional Communication Programs." *Technical Communication Quarterly* 23, no. 4, 2014, pp. 323–40, https://doi.org/10.1080/10572252.2014.942469.

Prentice, Rachel. *Bodies in Formation: An Ethnography of Anatomy and Surgery Education.* Duke UP, 2013.

Press, Sara. "The Politics of Standardized Patienthood." *Rhetoric of Health & Medicine* 5, no. 3, 2022, pp. 308–34, https://doi.org/10.5744/rhm.2022.50015.

Rajan-Rankin, Sweta. "Invisible Bodies and Disembodied Voices? Identity Work, the Body and Embodiment in Transnational Service Work." *Gender, Work, and Organization* 25, no. 1, 2018, pp. 9–23, https://doi.org/10.1111/gwao.12198.

Ratcliffe, Krista. *Rhetorical Listening: Identification, Gender, Whiteness*. Southern Illinois UP, 2005.

Rentmeester, Casey, and Meghan Liebzeit. "A Gadamerian Approach to Nursing: Merging Philosophy with Practice." *Nursing Philosophy* 24, no. 3, 2023, article e12453, pp. 1–7, https://doi.org/10.1111/nup.12453.

Rentmeester, Casey, et al. "Hermeneutical Healing: Physical Therapy with a Gadamerian Twist." *Journal of Applied Hermeneutics* 1, 2021, pp. 1–14.

Rifenburg, Michael J. *The Embodied Playbook: Writing Practices of Student-Athletes*. Utah State UP, 2018.

Rose, Mike. *The Mind at Work*. Penguin Books, 2005.

Rosen, Kathleen R. "The History of Medical Simulation." *Journal of Critical Care* 23, no. 2, 2008, pp. 157–66, https://doi.org/10.1016/j.jcrc.2007.12.004.

Roundtree, Aimee Kendall. *Computer Simulation, Rhetoric, and the Scientific Imagination: How Virtual Evidence Shapes Science in the Making and in the News*. Lexington Books, 2017.

Rowland, Allison L. *Zoetropes and the Politics of Humanhood*. The Ohio State UP, 2020.

Royster, Jacqueline Jones, and Gesa E. Kirsch. *Feminist Rhetorical Practices: New Horizons for Rhetoric, Composition, and Literacy Studies*. Southern Illinois UP, 2012.

Sahrmann, Shirley A. "The Human Movement System: Our Professional Identity." *Physical Therapy* 94, no. 12, 2014, pp. 1034–42, https://doi.org/10.2522/ptj.20130319.cx.

Sand-Jecklin, Kari, et al. "Video Monitoring for Fall Prevention and Patient Safety: Process Evaluation and Improvement." *Journal of Nursing Care Quality* 34, no. 2, 2019, pp. 145–50, https://doi.org/10.1097/NCQ.0000000000000355.

Sandelowski, Margarete. "Visible Humans, Vanishing Bodies, and Virtual Nursing: Complications of Life, Presence, Place, and Identity." *Advances in Nursing Science* 24, no. 3, 2002, pp. 58–70, https://doi.org/10.1097/00012272-200203000-00007.

Sauer, Beverly. "Embodied Experience: Representing Risk in Speech and Gesture." *Discourse Studies* 1, no. 3, 1999, pp. 321–54, https://doi.org/10.1177/1461445699001003003.

Sauer, Beverly. "Embodied Knowledge: The Textual Representation of Embodied Sensory Information in a Dynamic and Uncertain Material Environment." *Written Communication* 15, no. 2, 1998, pp. 131–69, https://doi.org/10.1177/0741088398015002001.

Schryer, Catherine F. "The Lab vs. the Clinic: Sites of Competing Genres." *Genre and the New Rhetoric*, edited by Aviva Freedman and Peter Medway, Taylor & Francis, 1994, pp. 105–24.

Selfe, Cynthia L., and Richard J. Selfe Jr. "The Politics of the Interface: Power and Its Exercise in Electronic Contact Zones." *College Composition and Communication* 45, no. 4, 1994, pp. 480–504, https://doi.org/10.2307/358761.

Selzer, Jack, and Sharon Crowley, eds. *Rhetorical Bodies*. U of Wisconsin P, 1999.

Shakespeare, Pam. "Nurses' Bodywork: Is There a Body of Work?" *Nursing Inquiry* 10, no. 1, 2003, pp. 47–56, https://doi.org/10.1046/j.1440-1800.2003.00158.x.

Siebers, Tobin. *Disability Theory*. U of Michigan P, 2008.

Singer, Ben. "The Human Simulation Lab—Dissecting Sex in the Simulator Lab: The Clinical Lacuna of Transsexed Embodiment." *Journal of Medical Humanities* 34, no. 2, 2013, pp. 249–54.

Siontis, Konstantinos C., et al. "Artificial Intelligence-Enhanced Electrocardiography in Cardiovascular Disease Management." *Nature Reviews Cardiology* 18, no. 7, 2021, pp. 465–78, https://doi.org/10.1038/s41569-020-00503-2.

Sloane, Todd. "Alarm Fatigue Solved by the AvaSure TeleSitter® Solution's Stat Alarm." *AvaSure*, 4 Dec. 2018, https://avasure.com/blog/alarm-fatigue-solved-by-the-avasure-telesitter-solutions-stat-alarm/.

Smith, Daniel L. "Intensifying Phronesis: Heidegger, Aristotle, and Rhetorical Culture." *Philosophy & Rhetoric* 36, no. 1, 2003, pp. 77–102, https://www.jstor.org/stable/40238138.

Spinuzzi, Clay. *Network: Theorizing Knowledge Work in Telecommunications.* Cambridge UP, 2008.

Spoel, Philippa, and Susan James. "The Textual Standardization of Midwives' Professional Relationships." *Discourse and Writing* 19, no. 1, 2003, pp. 3–29, https://doi.org/10.31468/cjsdwr.512.

Stafford, Trudi B., et al. "Working in an eICU Unit: Life in the Box." *Critical Care Nursing Clinics of North America* 20, no. 4, 2008, pp. 441–50, https://doi.org/10.1016/j.ccell.2008.08.013.

Stambler, Danielle. "Eating Data: The Rhetorics of Food, Medicine, and Technology in Employee Wellness Programs." *Rhetoric of Health & Medicine* 4, no. 2, pp. 158–86, https://doi.org/10.5744/rhm.2021.2003.

Strekalova, Yulia A., et al. "I Understand How You Feel: The Language of Empathy in Virtual Clinical Training." *Journal of Language and Social Psychology* 36, no. 1, 2017, pp. 61–79, https://doi.org/10.1177/0261927X16663255.

Stiller, Christine. "Exploring the Ethos of the Physical Therapy Profession in the United States: Social, Cultural, and Historical Influences and their Relationship to Education." *Journal of Physical Therapy Education*, 14, no. 3, 2000, pp. 7–16.

Sundén, Jenny. "Blonde Birth Machines: Medical Simulation, Techno-corporeality and Posthuman Feminism." *Technology and Medical Practice: Blood, Guts, and Machines*, edited by Ericka Johnson and Boel Berner, Ashgate Publishing, Ltd., 2010, pp. 97–117.

Swacha, Kathryn Yankura. "The Coping with COVID Project: Participatory Public Health Communication." *Communication Design Quarterly Review* 11, no. 1, 2023, pp. 4–18.

Tarr, Jennifer. "Educating with the Hands: Working on the Body/Self in Alexander Technique." *Sociology of Health & Illness* 33, no. 2, 2011, pp. 252–65, https://doi.org/10.1111/j.1467-9566.2010.01283.x.

Teston, Christa. *Bodies in Flux: Scientific Methods for Negotiating Medical Uncertainty.* U of Chicago P, 2017.

Topol, Eric. *Deep Medicine: How Artificial Intelligence Can Make Healthcare Human Again.* Hachette UK, 2019.

Trainor, Jennifer S. *Rethinking Racism: Emotion, Persuasion, and Literacy Education in an All-White High School.* Southern Illinois UP, 2009.

Twigg, Julia, et al. "Conceptualising Body Work in Health and Social Care." *Sociology of Health & Illness* 33, no. 2, 2011, pp. 171–88, https://doi.org/10.1111/j.1467-9566.2010.01323.x.

van den Broek, Diane. "Perforated Body Work: The Case of Tele-Nursing." *Work, Employment & Society: A Journal of the British Sociological Association* 31, no. 6, 2017, pp. 904–20, https://doi.org/10.1177/0950017016674899.

van Dongen, Els, and Riekje Elema. "The Art of Touching: The Culture of 'Body Work' in Nursing." *Anthropology & Medicine* 8, no. 2–3, 2001, pp. 149–62, https://doi.org/10.1080/13648470120101345.

Värri, Alpo, et al. "The Definition of Informatics Competencies in Finnish Healthcare and Social Welfare Education." *Digital Personalized Health and Medicine, Studies in Health Technology and Informatics*, edited by Louise B. Pape-Haugaard et al., 2020, pp. 1143–47.

Värri, Alpo Olavi, et al. "The National SotePeda 24/7 Project Develops Future Professional Competencies for the Digital Health and Social Care Sector in Finland." *Finnish Journal of EHealth and EWelfare* 11, no. 3, 2019, pp. 232–35, https://doi.org/10.23996/fjhw.77605.

Vee, Annette. "Large Language Models Write Answers." *Composition Studies* 51, no. 1, 2023, pp. 176–221.

Vidolov, Simeon, and Ivan Vidolov. "Understanding Virtual Embodiment: A Phenomenological Lens." *Proceedings of the 52nd Hawaii International Conference on System Sciences*, Hawaii International Conference on System Sciences, 2019, pp. 6500–508, http://hdl.handle.net/10125/60084.

Votruba, Lisbeth, et al. "Video Monitoring to Reduce Falls and Patient Companion Costs for Adult Inpatients." *Nursing Economics* 34, no. 4, 2016, pp. 185–89.

Wainwright, Emma, et al. "The Microgeographies of Learning Bodies and Emotions in the 'Classroom-Salon.'" *Emotion, Space and Society* 3, no. 2, 2010, pp. 80–89, https://doi.org/10.1016/j.emospa.2010.01.001.

Wang, Weiguang, et al. "Friend or Foe? The Influence of Artificial Intelligence on Human Performance in Medical Chart Coding." *SSRN*, 2019, https://doi.org/10.2139/ssrn.3405759.

Watson, Anne, et al. "Inpatient Nursing Care and Early Warning Scores: A Workflow Mismatch." *Journal of Nursing Care Quality* 29, no. 3, 2014, pp. 215–22, https://doi.org/10.1097/NCQ.0000000000000058.

Weaver, Amy. "High-Fidelity Patient Simulation in Nursing Education: An Integrative Review." *Nursing Education Perspectives* 32, no. 1, 2011, pp. 37–40.

Weedon, Scott, and T. Kenny Fountain. "Embodied Genres, Typified Performances, and the Engineering Design Process." *Written Communication* 38, no. 4, 2021, pp. 587–626, https://doi.org/10.1177/07410883211031508.

Wilson, Greg, and Carl G. Herndl. "Boundary Objects as Rhetorical Exigence: Knowledge Mapping and Interdisciplinary Cooperation at the Los Alamos National Laboratory." *Journal of Business and Technical Communication* 21, no. 2, 2007, pp. 129–54, https://doi.org/10.1177/1050651906297164.

Witman, Yolande. "What Do We Transfer in Case Discussions? The Hidden Curriculum in Medicine." *Perspectives on Medical Education* 3, no. 2, 2014, pp. 113–23, https://doi.org/10.1007/s40037-013-0101-0.

Wolkowitz, Carol. *Bodies at Work*. SAGE Publications, 2006.

Wolkowitz, Carol. "The Social Relations of Body Work." *Work, Employment and Society* 16, no. 3, 2002, pp. 497–510, https://doi.org/10.1177/095001702762217452.

Yam, Shui-Yin Sharon. *Inconvenient Strangers: Transnational Subjects and the Politics of Citizenship*. The Ohio State UP, 2019.

Yuan, H. Bin, et al. "The Contribution of High-Fidelity Simulation to Nursing Students' Confidence and Competence: A Systematic Review." *International Nursing Review* 59, no. 1, 2012, pp. 26–33.

INDEX

accreditation, 87, 122, 135
actants, 22, 83; bodies as, 23, 45; human, 42; nonhuman, 23, 83. *See also* intra-action
actor-network, 22
agential-realism, 23
alarm fatigue, 7, 125n2
Alexander Technique, 102
algorithms, 6–8, 161–62; and bias, 5, 8, 30, 127–28; and biometric data, 1, 8; and patient deterioration, 7, 130–31; provider attitudes toward, 7
anatomical knowledge, 29, 88, 95
anatomy labs. *See* dissection labs
Angeli, Elizabeth, 9, 13n4, 30, 130
apparatus, 23, 49
apprenticeship in nursing, 55–56
Arendt, Hannah, 20
Aristotle, 26
Artificial Intelligence (AI), 6–8, 161; and bias, 6; and diagnosis, 6–7; in tele-observation, 129–30. *See also* algorithms
assimilation: in physical therapy, 88; in simulations, 53, 83

Barad, Karen, 23
Barrows, Howard S., 56
Bawarshi, Anis, 23, 79
Bedor Hiland, Emma, 5, 128–29, 165
Benjamin, Ruha, 128

bias: in algorithms, 5, 8, 30, 127–28; in AI, 6
Blakenship, Lisa, 50
Bodies in Flux, 26–27, 29
body: Black male, 36–37; definitions of, 22–26; disability perspectives of, 18–19, 45; as event, 24–25; feminist perspectives of, 19; materialist perspectives of, 22–25; and metaphor, 24; nonnormative, 22, 83; optimization, 21; and private spaces, 18–19, 40–41; social constructionist perspectives of, 19. *See also* embodiment; embodied knowledge
body work, 8–11, 17, 45; and class, 17, 19, 21, 38–39; in classroom, 39, 58; cultural differences in, 38, 127; and gender, 8, 22, 35–40; Gimlin on, 2, 19; economics of, 8–9, 21; in healthcare, 30–35; in massage, 33–34, 87, 90, 113–14; in nursing, 8, 32, 49, 58, 70–71; physical impact of, 19, 157–59; in physical therapy, 33–34, 86–87; professional status and, 31, 33–34, 38–40, 87–90, 92–93, 102 (*see also* touch professions); racial hierarchies in, 9, 35–40, 166–67; sexualization and, 90, 92, 106 (*see also* sexualization); in sociology, 14, 17–19, 30–31, 35; technological mediation of, 15; in tele-observation, 34–35; Wolkowitz on, 2, 8–9, 19
boundaries, physical, 108, 112–14
boundary-work, 46, 162; embodied, 89–91, 93, 99–100, 123; patient stories as, 99–108; in physical therapy, 120; rhetorical, 88–89, 91, 122

195

Bourdieu, Pierre, 23, 29, 91. *See also* habitus
Britt, Elizabeth, 27, 42, 137
burnout, 34, 158–59, 167–68

call centers, embodiment in, 127, 138–39
capitalism, late-stage, 20–21
care work, 20, 44; versus body work, 17, 22; economic devaluing of, 20–21; global chains of, 37–38
catheter insertion, 58, 67, 71, 143, 151
certified nursing assistant (CNA), 135–38, 140, 148
certified nursing assistant (CNA) certification, 125n3, 132
charting: and body work, 10–11; in simulations, 60, 76–81; in tele-observation, 145–46; "to-do" list, 77–79. *See also* electronic health records; patient documentation; patient sense: charting and
ChatGPT, 163–64
Chávez, Karma, 22
Childish Gambino, 36–37
civic participation, 41, 44; and psycho-surveillance, 129
classroom: student relationships in, 110–12, 116; tacit knowledge in, 23–24, 28, 32, 42; visual learning in, 29, 55; versus workplace, 12, 39, 58, 84, 99, 136–38. *See also* collaboration: in classroom; educational contexts
collaboration: in classroom, 60, 108–9, 112–13; interdisciplinary, 13–14, 44, 168; interprofessional (*see* interprofessional communication); in virtual contexts, 126–27. *See also* tele-observation: collaboration and
Complementary and Alternative Medicine (CAM), 87–89, 123, 162
COVID-19, 90, 110, 131. *See also* telemedicine: and COVID-19
cues: discursive, 50, 83, 143, 162; environmental, 126–7; nonverbal, 117–18, 134, 136, 148 (*see also* gesture); from prior experience, 139–41, 143; sensory, 9, 30, 47, 71–72; technological, 68
cultural awareness, 4, 50, 81–85
cultural differences, 38; in simulations, 65–68, 81–85
cultural turn, 168; in sociology, 19, 22, 25

cyborg: body, 35; ontology, 35, 54, 164

data, 34, 68n2; biomedical emphasis on, 11, 45; intuition and, 29–30, 154–55, 159; and medical decision-making, 29, 142
debriefs: in nursing simulations, 4, 12–13, 60–62, 71, 80–81; as site for cultural learning, 84, 122, 166
deep acting, 51, 73
deep vein thrombosis, 69; creating clot for, 71–72; discovery of, 77–79
Derkatch, Colleen, 89
diagnosis, 87, 102, 136–37, 154; AI and, 6–7
disability, 24–25, 27, 41. *See also* simulations: disability in
discernment, 37
discourse, appropriation of, 40, 55
discourse analysis, multimodal, 2, 96
disruption, 14–15, 23, 31, 45, 164; definition of, 53; instructor-introduced, 53, 68–72; and manikin, 53–54, 68–73; in research, 44; in simulations, 50, 53–55. *See also* reflection: disruption and
dissection labs, 29, 55, 57, 115, 120
doctors. *See* physicians
domestic work, 37–38
Duckworth, Tammy, 41
Duggar, Patty, 56

educational contexts: habitus in, 12, 23, 25, 29, 91; informal, 46, 160; nontraditional, 126; online, 160, 163; power relations in, 12, 42, 44; as research site, 12, 23, 29, 42, 46. *See also* classroom
efficiency, 41, 77, 123
electrical stimulation, 86, 115, 118–20, 166, 168
electronic health records, 1, 6; access to, 142, 150–51, 153–54; and AI, 6, 161. *See also* charting; patient documentation
embodied knowledge, 24–30; class and, 38–39; gender and, 39–40; in legal education, 27, 137; in mining, 9–10, 26, 28, 39, 127 (*see also* pit sense); mothering and, 33, 39–40, 87, 90; patient documentation and, 76–81; of patients, 89–90, 105, 107–8, 121, 133; phronesis and, 26–27; race and, 35–38. *See also* body work; patient sense; phronesis; rhetorical body work

embodied learning, 24, 53, 68–73, 107–8, 109–17, 120

embodied rhetoric, 9–10, 22–25, 27–29, 40–42, 165. *See also* rhetorical body work

embodied writing, 41–42, 44

embodiment: complex, 25; differential, 113, 117–19, 121–22 (*see also* physical difference); virtual, 126–27

Emergency Medical Services (EMS), 9, 13n4. *See also* Angeli, Elizabeth

emotional distancing, 40, 67, 139, 148–50, 157, 167

emotional modulation: of nurses, 136; of patients, 81–83, 137, 139; of self, 37, 81–83, 106–8, 119, 121, 137, 150. *See also* laughter

empathy, 57; as body work, 50–52; critical, 54; interprofessional, 141; in nursing, 49; in patient communication (*see* patient communication: empathy and); rhetorical, 50–51; teaching of, 27, 46, 51, 64–67, 73–75, 136–37, 162

"Empathy Exams," 3n3, 56–57

energeia, 52

engineering experience: versus pit sense, 28–30; and writing, 41

ethnography, 13, 96, 163; and embodied presence, 41–44. *See also* fieldwork; interviews; observations; research

ethos, professional, 88, 90–91, 94

evidence: in biomedicine, 89; patient sense as, 150, 156

experiential learning, 55–58, 163

expertise, 9–11, 167; in physical therapy, 31–34, 86–87, 92–94, 101–2, 104–7, 123, 162; in tele-observation, 31, 126, 129, 153–54, 159

fall prevention, 128, 147

femininity: in massage therapy, 33, 39–40, 87, 90, 121–22; in midwifery, 89; in nursing, 40, 166; in physical therapy, 91–94, 166

feminism: apparent, 41, 119, 123; material, 44–45, 49

feminist: critiques of identification, 68 (*see also* identification); critiques of manikins, 48–49, 166; definitions of body, 35; rhetorical methods, 41–44; values in midwifery, 89

fieldwork, 2, 11–14, 95–96; rhetorical, 40–44, 168; power relations in, 42–43, 50. *See also* ethnography; interviews; observations; research

focal participants, 12–13, 134

focal students, 12–13, 62, 95

Foucault, Michel, 55, 59n1

Fountain, T. Kenny, 29, 55, 115, 120

Fraser, Nancy, 20

gaze, clinical, 55

gender: and body work, 8, 22, 35–40; and embodied knowledge, 39–40; and manikin, 4, 48, 59–60, 64–65, 83, 166; and physical therapy, 112–14; and rhetorical body work, 165–68; and simulations, 40, 48, 64; and trans embodiment, 83. *See also* femininity; masculinity

genre, 23–24; network, 24; patient medical form as, 79–80; prior knowledge of, 76

gesture, 10, 24, 38, 41–44. *See also* cues: nonverbal

Gieryn, Thomas, 88–89, 122

gig work, 129

Gimlin, Debra, 17, 19, 25, 51. *See also* body work

Graham, S. Scott, 6, 127–28, 161

habitus, 20, 23, 45, 91; empathetic, 51; professional, 25. *See also* Bourdieu, Pierre; educational contexts: habitus in

Haraway, Donna, 35, 164

Hawhee, Debra, 27

Hayles, Katherine, 126, 165

healthcare providers: in international contexts, 38, 165; precarity of, 16, 87, 129; training of, 4, 84–85. *See also* physicians

health insurance, 64, 158; claim investigation, 138–39; and professional status, 87, 89, 94 (*see also* accreditation)

Heidegger, Martin, 26, 59, 59n1

hidden curriculum, 15, 86–88, 90–91, 99–100, 120–22, 166–67

Hochschild, Arlie, 17, 37–38, 82. *See also* deep acting

holistic healthcare, 49, 90, 102–3, 121

humor, 82–83. *See also* laughter

identification: difference and, 54, 66–67; empathy and, 51–54, 66–67, 75 (see also empathy: teaching of); feminist critiques of, 68; in-group, 37, 107, 111–12; between instructor and manikin, 51, 72

immigrants and body work, 17, 36. See also body work: racial hierarchies in; care work: global chains of

incentive spirometers, race and, 127–28

informatics, materiality of, 126, 165

interprofessional communication, 7, 49, 88, 121, 141, 150–57, 159–60

intersectionality, 12, 36

interviews, 12, 62, 96, 126, 130–32; in sociology, 41

intra-action, 23–25, 29, 49, 54, 71–73, 75, 166–69. See also actants

intuition: in healthcare, 28, 30; in mining, 28–29; in professional communication, 9–10, 154; in tele-observation, 130, 154, 159–62

Jamison, Leslie, 3n3, 56–57

jargon, 135

Joslin, Eric, 61–63

Journal of the American Medical Association (JAMA), 89

Kerschbaum, Stephanie, 25

Kessler, Molly, 25

Knoblauch, Abby, 40

labor versus work, 20–21

Latour, Bruno, 22

laughter, 37, 71, 82, 111–12, 115–16, 118–20, 166

Lee, Jason, 61, 63–65, 69–72, 74–75, 77–83; and Chinese heritage, 81–83

LeMesurier, Jennifer, 24, 36–37

Lindquist, Julie, 51

listening, deep, 50–51

Magelssen, Scott, 37, 52, 82–83

manikin, 3–4, 57–60; crying, 74–75, 168; disruptions and, 53–54, 68–73; empathy and, 46, 52, 64–66, 73–75, 81–83, 162; gender and, 4, 48, 59–60, 64–65, 83, 166; intra-action and, 54, 71–73, 75, 166; patient sense and, 49–50, 58, 72–73, 83–84; for pelvic exam, 48, 55; race and, 4, 61, 64–65; voice, 48, 52, 57

Marx, Karl, 19–20

masculinity, 39–41; in physical therapy, 91–94, 113, 119–23, 166

materialist approach, 22–26, 73, 75–76; feminist, 44–45, 49

medical errors, 3n2, 6–7, 155–56

medical humanities, 51, 167. See also rhetoric: of health and medicine

medical terminology, 135. See also translanguaging; translation

Merleau-Ponty, Maurice, 29

metaphor, 77, 122, 141; somatic, 24

mêtis, 10, 27–28. See also phronesis

migration, 22. See also care work: global chains of

Milwaukee, WI, 36

movement system as domain of physical therapy, 90, 92, 94

Mulla, Sameena, 40, 76

"My Body on the Scene," 13, 42, 62–63, 98–99, 132–33

narrative: illness, 25, 50–52; inter-generational transmission of, 104, 107; morals in, 103; physical therapy patient, 104–7, 121; physical therapy provider, 103–4, 121; physical therapy origin, 99–103

neoliberal healthcare, 129

Noble, Sofiya Umoja, 128

nonverbal communication, 41–42. See also cues: nonverbal; gesture

Norris, Meriel, 33, 108, 113–14

Norris, Sigrid, 96

notes section, 10–11, 79–80, 145

novice-to-expert, 10, 28–29, 33, 55, 110

nursing: body work in, 8, 32, 49, 58, 70–71; empathy in, 49; history of, 55–56

objective information, 145

observations, 12–14, 36, 60–63, 95–97, 126, 130–31; in sociology, 41 optimism: about AI, 6, 161, 168; in physical therapy, 91–92, 94, 100

Osorio, Ruth, 41

pain thresholds in physical therapy practice, 111, 114–15, 117–20

patient actors, 3n3, 56–57

patient advocacy, 7, 40, 49, 53, 103–4

patient cameras, 132–33, 144, 148; removal of, 145, 152–53

patient communication: authority and, 146–47; cultural sensitivity and, 4, 81–83 (*see also* cultural differences: in simulations); empathy and, 15, 57, 64–65, 73–75, 81–83, 137–39, 161; impact of charting on, 77–81; intuition and, 130 (*see also* intuition: in professional communication); tailoring of, 119, 139, 146, 168; technology and, 1, 114–20, 146–47; touch and, 109–13; trust and, 31, 121; stereotyping and, 4, 121

patient discharge, 135

patient documentation, 23–24, 144–46; collection of, 13, 62; delays in, 7; embodied knowledge and, 76–81; emotional knowledge in, 79–80; teaching of, 76–81. *See also* charting; electronic health records; patient sense: charting and

patient experience: integration into care, 49, 79–80, 105, 137–38 (*see also* embodied knowledge: of patients); research emphasis on, 31–32, 133

patient hand-offs, 6, 62–63, 150–51; role of documentation in, 145

patient identities: Asian, 65, 81–83 (*see also* Lee, Jason); dementia, 147; elderly, 51–52, 64–66 (*see also* Ruiz, Eliana); with frontal lobe injury, 104, 141–42; Hispanic, 65 (*see also* Ruiz, Eliana); male, 67, 75; marginalized, 122, 166; multiple sclerosis, 56; schizophrenic, 137, 147; stroke victims, 98, 104, 129

patient preparation sheet, 50, 63–68, 83; images in, 64–66, 83

patient sense, 1–2, 9–11, 26–30, 45, 162–65, 167–69; and biomedical frameworks, 89, 123; charting and, 28, 76–81 (*see also* charting); communication of, 10–11; customer service and, 138–39; disruption and, 53, 83–85; expertise and, 11, 15, 105; in physical therapy lab, 86, 91, 103–5,

108–10, 116–17; in simulations, 49–50, 58, 63–65, 68, 72–73, 83–85, 162; technological mediation of, 11, 30, 45, 127, 155, 163–65; in tele-observation, 124–26, 133–43, 148, 155–57, 159–60, 162. *See also* embodied knowledge; pit sense; phronesis

patient sitting, 124, 128

patient-centered care, 90, 139; robots and, 14, 49

pedagogical contexts. *See* educational contexts

pediatrics, 62–63, 68–69, 80–81

phronesis, 2, 9–10, 26–27, 167; and disruption, 53–54, 164; and embodiment, 27–28; in healthcare, 9–10, 27–28, 45; versus mêtis (*see* mêtis). *See also* embodied knowledge; patient sense; pit sense

physical difference, 25, 36, 38, 64–65, 84, 112–22

physical technologies lab, 94–96, 108–9; marginalized groups in, 122

physical therapy: body work in, 33–34, 86–87; and diverse bodies, 113, 121–22; gender and, 112–14 (*see also* femininity: in physical therapy; masculinity: in physical therapy); history of, 91–94; narrative in (*see* narrative); versus personal training, 33–34; physical moves of, 109–14; positive attitude of, 91–92, 94, 100–101; professional identity, 90, 104, 121–23; relationship to technology, 93–94, 108–9, 114–20, 166; rigor of, 101; sexualization of, 90, 92, 106, 113–14, 122; verbal interaction in, 109–20

physicians: physical therapists versus, 93, 102–4, 107; research emphasis on, 31, 133, 163, 167

physician's orders, 70, 73, 76–77

pit sense, 2, 9–10, 26–32, 45, 54, 107; and writing, 28. *See also* Sauer, Beverly

pity versus empathy, 52, 57

polio epidemic influence on physical therapy, 91–92, 94

posthumanism, 34; Barad on, 23; Latour on, 22

precarity of healthcare providers, 16, 87, 129

Prentice, Rachel, 54–55

Press, Sara, 3–4, 56, 83, 122

private sphere. *See* public sphere

professional experience, 125, 133–34, 138–43, 163

professional identity, 82–83, 86, 91, 120, 162; and narrative, 99–108, 121–22 (*see also* narrative); and objects, 28–29, 115, 120

professional history: of nursing, 55–56; of physical therapy, 91–94

professional status, 21–22, 25–26, 31–35, 87; of midwifery, 89, 104; of nursing, 55–56; of physical therapy, 88–94, 102–3, 106–7

professionalism: and femininity, 40, 88, 90–94, 120–22, 166 (*see also* femininity; masculinity); and social barriers, 33–34

programmed patient. *See* patient actors; standardized patients

public sphere, 40–41. *See also* workplace context

pulse oximeters, 131n1; race and, 8, 127–28

race: embodied knowledge and, 35–38; hierarchies in body work, 9, 35–40, 166–67; incentive spirometers and, 127–28; kinesiology of, 36–37; manikin and, 4, 61, 64–65; pulse oximeters and, 8, 127–28; rhetorical body work and, 165–68; simulations and, 64; tele-observers and, 133–34, 166; in virtual contexts, 127–28

Ratcliffe, Krista, 43, 75

reflection, 12, 24; critical, 26–27, 53, 163–64; disruption and, 15, 50, 53, 73, 84–85

research, 40–44; access, 13–14; consent, 12–13; ethics, 12–13; and positionality, 13, 42–43, 60; questions, 11. *See also* ethnography; fieldwork

rhetoric: embodied (*see* cues: nonverbal; embodied rhetoric; gesture; nonverbal communication); of health and medicine, 31, 163, 168–69 (*see also* medical humanities); material, 14, 18, 22–23, 165 (*see also* body: materialist perspectives of; feminism: material; informatics, materiality of; materialist approach); visual, 29 (*see also* trained vision)

rhetorical body work, 1–2, 8–11, 44–47, 161–63, 167–69; definition of, 17, 44; discursive, 45, 63–68, 76–81, 111, 147; emotional, 26, 64, 73–75, 81–83, 107, 161; gender and, 165–68; and miscommunication, 80–81; in nursing simulations, 50, 81; physical, 26, 68–73, 123, 127; in physical therapy lab, 99, 102, 108–20; race and, 165–68; teaching of, 26, 72–73, 105–8; in tele-observation, 15, 124–26, 134, 143–44, 150, 157, 159–60

rhetorical education, 27, 42, 160; in ancient Greece, 27

rhetorical enactments, 25

rhetorical listening, 43, 75

rhetorical skills: higher-order, 37–38, 152; lower-order, 38–39

rhetorical style, 89

robots, 168; in mining, 54, 127; in simulations, 1, 3–4, 57–58, 83–84, 166; voice, 136, 146–47. *See also* manikin

Rose, Mike, 39

Rothman Index, 7–8, 30, 130–31

Roundtree, Aimee Kendall, 52

routinization, 23, 39; and disruption, 53–54

Rowland, Allison, 35–36

Ruiz, Eliana, 61, 64–66, 71

Sanderson, Marguerite, 92

Sauer, Beverly, 2, 9–10, 26–32, 45, 127. *See also* pit sense

scientific knowledge: curricular emphasis on, 33, 40; in physical therapy, 87, 120 (*see also* expertise: in physical therapy; movement system as domain of physical therapy); in relation to pit sense, 9, 29–30. *See also* technical knowledge

sequential compression devices (SCDs), 72, 72n4, 77–79

sexualization, 33, 40, 56, 87, 90, 106–8; of body work, 90, 92, 106; of physical therapy, 90, 92, 106, 113–14, 122

Siebers, Tobin, 24, 52

sim stupor, 60–63

simisms, 60, 71, 80

SimMan, 3–4, 57

SimOne, 57

simulation coordinator, 48, 59–60, 68–69; cultural knowledge, 81, 83–84; embodied immersion, 72, 84–85. *See also* disruption: instructor-introduced

simulation lab, 58–63, 68–69

simulations: critical, 52–53; disability in, 52; disruption in, 50–55; fidelity in, 48–50,

54, 71–72; gender and, 40, 48, 64; in health education, 3–4, 48–49; in nursing, 40, 48–49, 57–58, 60–63; race and, 64. *See also* manikin; patient actors; standardized patients

social constructionist lens, 23; of the body, 19, 21

sociology: and body/work nexus, 17, 18–19; methods, 41. *See also* body work: in sociology; cultural turn: in sociology

SotePeda 24/7, 165

standardized care, 87, 89

standardized patients, 3–4, 55–58; and cultural knowledge, 83; and empathy, 57; and personality, 56. *See also* patient actors

stat alarm, 125n2, 136, 146–47, 149

stereotyping, 91; patient communication and, 4, 121; patients, 50, 83, 88, 119–22, 166; providers, 167

story. *See* narrative

subjective information, 90, 145

Sundén, Jenny, 4

surface acting, 51–52, 73

tacit knowledge, 12, 30, 32, 41; in classroom, 23–24, 28, 32, 42

task-oriented, 73; charting, 77–79

technical knowledge, 33, 40, 129, 163; and phronesis, 53. *See also* scientific knowledge

technological mediation, 1, 18; in education, 164–65; embodied knowledge and, 167–68; and habitual action, 163–64 (*see also* disruption; technology: and disruption); and patient sense, 11, 30, 45, 127, 155, 163–65; in tele-observation, 15, 124–25, 150

technology: and attention, 115–17, 120; and disruption, 54, 132–33, 164 (*see also* disruption); and healthcare access, 128; and physical difference, 117–20, 127–28 (*see also* physical difference)

telehealth, 1, 4–6, 8, 160; critiques of, 5–6; and patient monitoring, 5

telemedicine, 4–6; and COVID-19, 5, 8, 128 (*see also* COVID-19); and mental healthcare (*see* teletherapy)

telemetry, 68n2, 155

tele-nursing, 34, 126–27; relationship to tele-observers, 142, 153

tele-observation, 124–25; collaboration and, 129, 157, 159–60; and customer service, 138–39; history of, 128–30; listening and, 152; marginalization of, 15, 129, 145–46, 159–60, 166–67; patient protocols in, 125, 152; physical toll of, 149–50, 157–59, 167

tele-observers, 131–32; age and, 142; documentation and, 125, 142–46, 150–51, 156, 160, 167; emotional investment of, 142, 148–50 (*see also* emotional distancing); formal education of, 136–38, 154; healthcare experience of, 140–43; onboarding of, 134–36, 147; organizational strategies of, 143–46; race and, 133–34, 166; relationship to nurses, 125, 136–37, 141, 143, 149–57; relationship to patients, 136–37, 143–50; trust in, 153–56; use of redirects, 125, 135, 146–47; volunteers as, 129n1

tele-sitting. *See* tele-observation; tele-observers

teletherapy, 5, 128–29, 165

teleworkers, 126–28; relationship with hospital staff, 6–7, 150–57; trust in, 153–54. *See also* tele-observation; tele-observers

Teston, Christa, 26–29

Topol, Eric, 161

touch professions, 15, 45, 87, 123. *See also* body work: professional status and

trained vision, 29, 55

Trainor, Jennifer, 91

transfer of care. *See* patient hand-offs

transgender embodiment, 83

translanguaging, 38. *See also* medical terminology; translation

translation, 43, 45, 52, 76. *See also* medical terminology; translanguaging

ultrasound, 72, 77, 86, 115–17

uniforms, 25, 33, 90

video recording, 13, 61–62, 95–97, 130; as disruptive, 44

virtual intensive care unit (VICU), 124–26, 130–33; physical experience of, 142, 149–50, 157–59

virtual workplace, 126–28

vital signs, 57, 60, 68, 71

Wainwright, Emma, 33, 39–40, 90, 108, 113–14, 121–22
wellness technology, 8, 36
Wolkowitz, Carol, 2, 17–22, 25, 161; and cultural turn, 19, 22, 25; and marginalized work, 2, 35, 45, 87; and paid work, 21, 44; and professional status, 31, 90, 102. *See also* body work

work: blue-collar, 38–39 (*see also* working class); in democratic market-based economies, 21–22; invisible, 35–36, 45; versus labor, 20–21; white-collar, 21, 38–39, 93, 160
working class, 19, 38–39, 156, 160
workplace contexts, 7–9, 12, 40–41, 82; prior experience in (*see* professional experience)
World War II, women's role during, 93n1

NEW DIRECTIONS IN RHETORIC AND MATERIALITY
ALLISON L. ROWLAND, CHRISTA TESTON, AND SHUI-YIN SHARON YAM,
SERIES EDITORS

Current conversations about rhetoric signal ongoing attentiveness to and critical appraisal of material-discursive phenomena. New Directions in Rhetoric and Materiality provides a forum for responding to and extending such conversations, but also asks that books published in the series attend to social events of consequence unfolding around the world—such as violence based on misinformation, continued police brutality, immigration legislation and migration crises, and more. The series therefore seeks to amplify books that examine rhetoric's relationship to materiality while also confronting material-rhetorical forces of oppression, power imbalances, and differential vulnerabilities.

Patient Sense: Rhetorical Body Work in the Age of Technology
  LILLIAN CAMPBELL

Trafficking Rhetoric: Race, Migration, and the Making of Modern-Day Slavery
  ANNIE HILL

Nuclear Decolonization: Indigenous Resistance to High-Level Nuclear Waste Siting
  DANIELLE ENDRES

Decolonial Conversations in Posthuman and New Material Rhetorics
  EDITED BY JENNIFER CLARY-LEMON AND DAVID M. GRANT

Untimely Women: Radically Recasting Feminist Rhetorical History
  JASON BARRETT-FOX

Violent Exceptions: Children's Human Rights and Humanitarian Rhetorics
  WENDY S. HESFORD

Zoetropes and the Politics of Humanhood
  ALLISON L. ROWLAND

Ecologies of Harm: Rhetorics of Violence in the United States
  MEGAN EATMAN

Raveling the Brain: Toward a Transdisciplinary Neurorhetoric
  JORDYNN JACK

Post-Digital Rhetoric and the New Aesthetic
  JUSTIN HODGSON

Not One More! Feminicidio on the Border
  NINA MARIA LOZANO

Visualizing Posthuman Conservation in the Age of the Anthropocene
  AMY D. PROPEN

Precarious Rhetorics
  EDITED BY WENDY S. HESFORD, ADELA C. LICONA, AND CHRISTA TESTON

www.ingramcontent.com/pod-product-compliance
Lightning Source LLC
Chambersburg PA
CBHW020732240426
43665CB00052B/456